T0068412

Unraveling the Mystery of

AUTISM

and Pervasive

Developmental Disorder

———

A Mother's Story of
Research and Recovery

———

KARYN SEROUSSI

Simon & Schuster Paperbacks
New York London Toronto Sydney New Delhi

Simon & Schuster Paperbacks
A Division of Simon & Schuster, Inc.
1230 Avenue of the Americas
New York, NY 10020

This Simon & Schuster trade paperback edition October 2014

SIMON & SCHUSTER PAPERBACKS and colophon are registered trademarks of Simon & Schuster, Inc.

For information about special discounts for bulk purchases, please contact Simon & Schuster Special Sales at 1-866-506-1949 or business@simonandschuster.com.

The Simon & Schuster Speakers Bureau can bring authors to your live event. For more information or to book an event contact the Simon & Schuster Speakers Bureau at 1-866-248-3049 or visit our website at www.simonspeakers.com.

Interior design by Jill Putorti
Cover photograph by Teresa A. Kerr

Manufactured in the United States of America

10   9   8   7   6   5   4   3   2   1

Library of Congress Cataloging-in-Publication Data is available.

ISBN 978-1-4814-2944-3
ISBN 978-1-4391-4262-2 (ebook)

TO FRANK MCCOURT, my dearest teacher, who always told me that someday I would have something important to write about. Before you were an inspiration to millions, you were an inspiration to me. Thank you for giving me the skills I needed so that when the day came, I was able to do the job.

TO MY HUSBAND, ALAN, who is the most brilliant and beautiful man I know.

TO MY MOTHER, RISHA, who always made me believe I could do anything.

TO PAUL SHATTOCK, who defines the word "generosity." Without his timely interference, I do not believe my son would have gotten better. Paul was not just in the right place at the right time; he was in the right place for a long time, and that has made all the difference in hundreds and hundreds and hundreds of lives.

Acknowledgments

I gratefully acknowledge Lisa Lewis for her enormous contribution to the widespread use of dietary intervention for the treatment of autism. Lisa is not only my greatest resource for cooking help, but a valued friend, and she shines as one of the good things in my life that have come out of the autism experience.

I would also like to thank my wonderful children for giving up so much time with their mommy so that I could research and write this book. With her usual wisdom, Laura says it made her understand how important it is to help others when they need us.

Thanks to my amazing sister Jessica and exceptional brothers Matthew and Eric, to Howard Shaw and my mother, Risha Granat Shaw, to the wonderful Eileen Monastersky, and to my dear friends Stephanie and Kevin Kelly, all of whom gave me a place to write, read my drafts, and gave lots of support and unconditional love. Thanks also to Dr. Richard Seroussi and Dr. Sylvia Seroussi, who replaced the lost branch of my family tree just when I needed it most, and to Jill Pavone for her cottage, her special ed skills, and her friendship.

Substantial appreciation goes to my agent, Kathi Paton, who listened and gave the best advice; to Roz Siegel at Simon & Schuster; and to Wayne Gilpin of Future Horizons, who apparently cares more about helping people with autism than about money.

Thanks also go to Dr. Jaak Panksepp, for proposing a far-fetched theory that turned out to be true; to Dr. Kalle Reichelt, at the University of Norway, for his gentle persistence; to Paul Shattock at the University of Sunderland in the United Kingdom for carrying the torch so selflessly and gracefully; to Dr. Andrew Wakefield at the Royal Free Hospital in London (who forgives me for being pushy); and to Dr. Alan Friedman, at Johnson & Johnson's Ortho Clinical Diagnostics, for believing me, and for finding what I prefer to believe will lead to the cure for autism.

I am also very grateful to Dr. Bernard Rimland of the Autism Research Institute in San Diego, for crusading tirelessly for so many families who needed him.

I would like to thank Lori Scime, Terri Kerr, Lori Ross, Mary Cropley, Jean Curtin, and Shari Rogers for their support and advice, and to give special thanks to Kathy Terrillion for her help and for all that she has done.

Thanks also to Jack Daiss, Ph.D., and Michelle Ray, also of Johnson & Johnson's Ortho Clinical Diagnostics; Dr. Susan Hyman and Dr. Mary Beth Robinson; to Dr. Robert Sinaiko, William Shaw, Ph.D., and Terence Hines, Ph.D.

Contents

Foreword

by Bernard Rimland, Ph.D.

Karyn Seroussi has written a superb, landmark book that will be of immense interest to everyone—especially those concerned with autistic children. On a scale of 1 to 10, I would rate *Unraveling the Mystery of Autism and Pervasive Developmental Disorder* a perfect 10. Why so high? The book is a multifaceted work, and each facet is a gem in itself.

Although this book reads like a gripping detective story, it is an all too true account of a brilliant mother's successful struggle to rescue her child from a "hopeless" disease. Her journey is our journey, as she takes us step by step on her voyage through the dark and mysterious world of autism.

What she discovers, over and over, is that conventional thinking about autism's nature, causes, and treatment is wrong—dreadfully wrong. By studying the medical literature, networking with researchers and other parents on the Internet, and brainstorming with her exceptionally astute scientist husband, she also discovers real solutions for her son's terrifying malady. In fact, she finds what all parents hope for: a cure for her son.

Karyn Seroussi's formerly autistic son is doing beautifully. I have met him—a charming, playful, creative youngster. Many other formerly autistic youngsters whose parents have adopted similar approaches are also doing beautifully. You will meet some of them, and their families, in the pages of Karyn's book. In addition, you will find specific detailed information that can make a lifesaving difference to children at all points on the autistic spectrum—from autism, through pervasive developmental disorder (PDD) and Asperger's syndrome (AS), to so-called attention deficit hyperactivity disorder (ADHD). Some of these children, like Karyn's, can be cured. Others can make astonishing progress, achieving far more than their parents ever dreamed was possible. Whether or not you have an autistic child, much of what you learn may also bring about unexpected health benefits to you and your family.

I am very well acquainted with the path Karyn Seroussi has so carefully mapped for today's parents. I began to explore that path in 1958, when my wife and I diagnosed our severely affected two-year-old son as autistic. (Our highly competent pediatrician had never seen nor heard of an autistic child in his thirty-five years of practice. I was five years beyond my Ph.D. in psychology when I first saw the word "autism.") In those days autism was thought to be a hopeless, incurable, emotional disorder brought on by unloving ("refrigerator") mothers. My book *Infantile Autism,* published in 1964, is credited with having destroyed that pernicious theory, and stimulated the search for biological causes.

Within a few years of my book's publication, I had heard from hundreds of parents of autistic children. From those letters and phone calls I became familiar with the elements of the story that Karyn Seroussi tells so well in this book. I heard from parents who *knew* that a vaccination had caused their children's autism, despite the fervent assertions of the medical establishment that the vaccines could do no harm. I heard from parents that they had tried high-dose vitamin therapy (especially vitamin B$_6$), often with excellent results, despite their doctors' insistence that vitamins could not possibly help. I heard from parents that their children improved amazingly upon being placed on a milk- or wheat-free diet, despite extreme skepticism from their doctors, who had never heard of a "food allergy" that could affect the brain. I began a decades-long struggle to resolve the discrepancy between these consistent parent observations and the sacred-cow beliefs of the medical establishment.

In 1972, I was invited to give a talk at the annual conference of the Autism Society of America (then called the National Society for Autistic Children). I discussed my research on the value of vitamin B$_6$ in autism and mentioned milk and wheat intolerances as possible causes of some cases of autism. "While I recognize that most physicians today are skeptical about such 'allergies of the nervous system,'" I had the audacity to suggest, "and that many have never heard the term, I will predict that in ten to fifteen years the average physician will think of such allergies as an immediate possibility when he sees an autistic-type child, or one with learning disabilities or hyperkinesis. Or, for that matter, an adult with migraine."

My guess that it would take ten to fifteen years for the medical establishment to become enlightened about food intolerance was obviously far too optimistic. Deeply entrenched views do not change quickly. But Karyn Seroussi's book will surely hasten the day when my prediction finally does come true.

What has changed in the nearly three decades since then? Nothing—and everything. *Nothing* has changed for those who accept the belief that psychotropic drugs, all of which pose significant risks, are the only worthwhile biomedical intervention for autism. *Everything* has changed for parents like Karyn, who pursue all promising avenues, often with excellent results. Dozens of published studies have revealed that milk and wheat proteins are culprits in many cases of autism—yet only a handful of doctors are aware of these studies.

A growing body of scientific research shows a strong link between autism and vaccination, most recently with the MMR (measles, mumps, rubella) vaccine—yet most doctors still scoff at the idea that immunization is a factor in autism. And eighteen consecutive studies, in six different countries, have shown that vitamin B_6 can be of enormous benefit to many autistic children—yet poorly informed doctors still tell parents that "vitamins have been shown to be useless."

Karyn Seroussi's book not only tells us much about autism, it also tells us a great deal about the need to take responsibility for our health and for the health of our children. We live in a world where respected physicians can be poorly informed, and all too often give inadequate advice.

Thus, in addition to being a truly interesting and inspiring personal story, *Unraveling the Mystery of Autism and Pervasive Developmental Disorder* confers an unexpected benefit to the general reader. This book offers an introduction to food intolerances as a very pervasive and all too often overlooked factor in human health.

Scientific research has only just begun to reveal the mechanisms behind the serious consequences that many people suffer as a result of unrecognized intolerances to certain foods. We have all heard the old saying "One man's meat is another man's poison," but few of us have recognized the wide-ranging implications of that wise observation. Karyn Seroussi's story will lead you to appreciate the relevance of that ancient adage to your well-being, and the well-being of those you care for.

The salient message of this book is that parents who want to help their autistic children must look beyond traditional medicine for answers. Effective treatments *are* available—far better treatments than merely drugging autistic children with psychotropic medications—but you are not likely to learn about these treatments from your child's doctor. You *will* learn about them, however, in the pages of this book. The information Karyn discovered on her journey has led to dramatic improvement, and sometimes even cures, in many autistic children. Now, thanks to *Unraveling the Mystery of Autism and Pervasive Developmental Disorder,* this crucial information will benefit thousands more. If you are the parent of an autistic child, I hope your son or daughter is among them.

Unraveling the Mystery of

AUTISM

and Pervasive

Developmental Disorder

Introduction

"Your book reads like a suspense novel, but it was even more chilling because it's true, and because it was so eerily similar to our daughter's story. I literally couldn't put it down."

—*Bill P. Sykes, Los Angeles*

"After the diagnosis ('D-Day,' as I call it), I didn't have the strength to read much about autism. But you have a gift for storytelling that had me on the edge of my seat, and the result of these interventions has been miraculous for my son. Thank goodness for your book—if we had waited for our doctor to tell us what to do, we'd be living with a very different child."

—*Susan Leach, New York*

"So many experiences, ideas, and beliefs you shared in your book matched everything I've been through in the past few months."

—*Kirsten Martinez, Miami, Florida*

"Your beautifully written book is a challenge to the medical community to listen to what their patients are telling them. Your stunning revelations will doubtless change the outcome for countless children claimed by what has become a tragic epidemic."

—*Heather Snyder, Pennsylvania*

"A book like this on autism has been long overdue. Now nobody can say he or she didn't know."

—*A parent in New Jersey*

I recently reread my book *Unraveling the Mystery of Autism and Pervasive Developmental Disorder* with a sense of amazement. It hardly seems possible that I wrote this book at all. Only a parent who is obsessed and overwhelmed by her child's special needs could create a work like that. I hope I never have a reason to write such a book again!

I am also amazed by the response to this book from the autism community. I have been told it effectively marks a watershed between the old belief that every case of autism is hardwired and incurable, and the new understanding that many cases are biologically treatable. My goal was to help parents feel empowered and be motivated to seek out answers for their children, and I am proud to hear that so many have. Instead of simply imitating my son's treatment protocol, many parents have become inspired to look further into their own children's individual biological profiles, and have broken new ground in the investigation of other metabolic and immunological issues leading to autistic disorders.

Luckily, thousands of children besides my son *have* had a dramatic response to the very treatments I describe. Most gratifying have been the letters I've received from parents who discovered these treatments in my book. The old cliché about self-help books is that "if just one person is helped, it's worthwhile." When it comes to the gluten- and dairy-free diet, thousands of children have been helped while waiting for medical science to catch up, thanks to the courageous and noble efforts of the many doctors, researchers, and parents who have taken up this cause.

I am often asked how my son is doing—"Is he still okay?" Yes, he is. He is strictly gluten- and dairy-free by choice, after a few accidental and unpleasant slipups over the years. He's well liked, good-natured, offbeat, philosophical, messy, absentminded: a little bit like his dad, and a little bit like his mom. In high school he got good grades despite an ongoing wrangle with inattention, participated avidly in concert choir and musical theater, and dabbled in writing fantasy fiction. He's had a couple of girlfriends. He has trouble deciding on a college major. I guess he struggles no more than the average nineteen-year-old.

That so many young people like him have now achieved normal functioning is evidence that, in the early stages of regressive autism, the disorder can be reversible. Miles is not the only child for whom the removal of opiate peptides from the diet led to a complete resolution of the autistic behaviors. Not a "cure," mind you, because the underlying cause of the disorder is still unknown, and the overlapping subtypes mean that some children may only be *helped* by the diet, but not recovered by it. Miles still has the disorder that causes autism. Treating it early on must have been a critical factor for him.

But so many doctors are still woefully uninformed about the new theories about autism's causes and treatments. Many are unwilling even to discuss these simple, safe interventions with their patients' parents, and often the parents have been made to feel like renegades. Some have even been accused of "child abuse" for doing something as simple as removing cow's milk from their children's diets. It is not in a child's best interest for the parent-doctor partnership of trust and open communication to be weakened.

I wish I could say that medical science has already caught up with our theories, but at least these things *are* moving ahead, albeit at a slow and steady pace. A revolution takes place only when the old system is proven to be unsatisfactory. For decades, our understanding and treatment of autism have been a terrible source of frustration for parents and professionals alike. Now, one success story after another has convinced a great number of people to stand up and take notice. A true paradigm shift in our global view of autism will take place, but it could take several more years of carefully designed studies and serious investigation before we can understand exactly why the diet and other "alternative" treatments are effective, and for which children they are appropriate.

I would also like to emphasize something very important: treatment for autism has to be multimodal. Foremost, if possible, take away the *cause* of the disorder and treat the underlying biological problems. There are many reasons why well-meaning parents resist this, including opposition from their doctors, which can be hard to overcome.

I'm sure to rub people the wrong way when I criticize those who won't try the diet, but right now we just don't know for certain which autistic kids need to be on it. From my perspective, it is heartbreaking to think of the children like my son, whose autistic behaviors are being *caused* by these proteins, who are suffering damage at every meal by loving parents unwilling to take the plunge.

One month after the first edition of this book came out, Lisa Lewis phoned me and said, "Karyn, we are getting fourteen hundred e-mails a week, and my fax machine is ringing nonstop. How the heck are we going to handle this? Are we really going to answer all this mail?"

Amazingly, we did. Over the next year we read over sixteen thousand e-mails, and answered every one. Most could not be answered with a form letter, as they were specific to each child. We did this as volunteers, and at times it was exhausting and frustrating. But it was also incredibly rewarding. To hear of the impact of our work on so many families was very powerful, and many times we found ourselves moved to tears by the letters we received.

Here are some typical responses I received from parents who had success with the diet:

"We recently celebrated the four-month anniversary of our son being a casein-free, gluten-free eater, and have noticed some remarkable changes. He is making excellent eye contact, has quite a bit of interest in his brother (where there was none), has made a huge improvement in receptive language, has introduced some verbal language, has improved sleep, less 'stimming,' less tantrumming, and is better able to handle public places and outings. He will now give kisses and hugs, and wave and say 'bye' (often without prompting!). Although I see such a need for further improvement, he is making progress very quickly. I feel confident that the improvement will continue, and for that I am forever grateful. We invited twenty-three people to our home to celebrate his second birthday. The fact that we were able to do this, and he was able to handle this, is quite remarkable. Before the diet, he would never have been able to handle that many people in our home."

—*Shelli Clarke, Erie, Pennsylvania*

"My four-year-old son could not say 'yes' or 'no' or address me as 'Mummy'—he had some basic echolalia only. He was very miserable and cried often. Sound sensitivities and gravitational issues were a problem, too. We started the gluten-free, casein-free diet five months ago, and instantly his red ears (which he had had for two years) disappeared. He lost the perpetual gray pallor. His picky eating habits persisted for two weeks, after which he ate everything I put in front of him! The sound and gravity problems are almost gone. He has gained eighteen months' worth of language in five months. He is so happy now, particularly when he looks me in the eyes and says, 'I have the prettiest mummy ever.' His advances are astounding his therapists, considering the late start to intervention. I feel (at last) confident for his future."

—*Lisa Andersen, Australia*

"I could shout from the highest mountain—Sam's progress continues to amaze us. He's getting closer all the time. This morning he came out of his room and said, 'Good morning, Mommy, how are you today?'"

—*Teresa Summers*

"He will give us kisses and hugs upon request, will get his shoes when asked, he is starting to point, he shakes his head yes or no, is always wanting to reach out and play with other children, and waits in line patiently. I truly believe if I had not started the diet when I did, I would have lost my son. Thank you."

—*A parent*

"In the few short weeks we have been doing the diet he is more social and empathetic. He spontaneously shares with his baby sister. He was so worried about my dad, who fell and hit his head on some cement stairs last week, that he wanted to call and talk to him every day (since now he will actually converse a little on the phone!), and the biggest thing is he is so much better at coping with life's little disappointments. The tantrums have drastically diminished, almost vanished."

—*Suzanne Dunford*

"Around here, the diet is looked upon as something that does not work, and doctors discourage parents from trying. I have living, *talking* proof that it does work."

—*Jody Goddard, Ellettsville, Indiana*

"My son is doing absolutely beautifully. We started the diet just over three months ago, at the end of October, and found out about his other food allergies the day before Thanksgiving. Since then, he has been gluten-free/casein-free as well as off all of the other twelve foods to which he is allergic. He started talking right after Christmas. He is two years and four months old, and his receptive language is now at or above age level. He follows almost all of our directions, and he is so eager to please. He does interlocking puzzles, has learned the alphabet, calls me 'Mommy,' plays with his toys (especially his choochoo trains), and has some pretend play. He is starting to put two words together: 'help me,' 'bye Mommy,' 'more (whatever).' His eye contact is getting better and better, and he is noticing other children. His ABA [applied behavior analysis] consultant can't get over his progress, and tells me each week that he is learning faster than she can believe. She also thinks that at this point he is off the autism spectrum. He still has some perseverations, although they are so minor, and I am always able to get him focused on to something more fun. In fact, he no longer opens and shuts doors, which was his main perseveration. He looks great (no more dark circles under his eyes), and his teachers at our 'Mommy and Me' class can't get over the change in him—he does all of the hand movements to the songs in class and 'sings' some of the words to our little songs. We are absolutely amazed by his progress."

—*A parent*

"We did not hear about this diet from any of the doctors or educators dealing with our son over the last four years. It wasn't until we read your story in *Parents* magazine that I was introduced to this subject. That night I stayed up all night, disposing of my entire kitchen. My husband got up at 5:30 A.M. to take a shower and found me in the middle of piles of boxes to donate to the homeless shelter. He asked what I was doing, and I explained that I was getting rid of all the food, spices, etc., in our house, and I showed him the 'safe' food list I had downloaded hours earlier. (I think he thought I had lost it, but with a smile he said it sounded like a great idea.) That was six months ago, and we can't believe the changes we have seen."

—*Stacey Solar, Belleair, Florida*

"We still have a lot of work to do, but we have so much *hope*. That 'knife' in my stomach is gone! The other day we were looking at a video and he leaned his head on mine. Then he turned and looked at me (and I looked at him) and he kissed me gently on the cheek. He didn't have to say anything at that moment, because I understood exactly what he was thinking."

—*Marie, San Jose, California*

Other nonbiological interventions such as special ed schools, speech therapy, and occupational therapy are *essential* for teaching the social and academic skills the child has missed, or cannot learn in typical ways.

I would also like to make something very clear. There is a great deal of debate about what kind of therapy is "best." My experience is that a parent *must* research the treatments and make the decision based on his or her knowledge of the child. Not because it worked well for my child or a friend's child, not because it's offered locally, not because it's cheaper or easier or more convenient. ABA, AIT, Son-Rise, other therapies . . . each has helped certain kids achieve their potential for growth and improvement.

You might hear some generalizations that may be useful. I have heard that ABA works really well for high-functioning kids and diet responders. Conversely, I've been told that Son-Rise Program (Option Institute) may be the gentlest, least invasive way of enlisting the cooperation of kids who are highly sensory-defensive and who make gains slowly. Some people say that Greenspan works best in conjunction with other therapies. There are simply no hard-and-fast rules. Trust your instincts. Use whatever makes sense and seems to work.

Some programs may not be fully compatible with each other, but elements of each can be used together. My son soared with ABA, but for some kids I knew, the intensity of the program seemed invasive and downright unkind. If, after several months, your child still bursts into tears at the sight of the therapist, you may need to rethink your choices.

Many people ask me whether I believe their child is too old for the diet. If you think about it, what they are really asking is if their child is too old for "recovery." In severely affected older children, teenagers, and adults, it is probably true that the chance of a totally "normal" life becomes slimmer as the years pass. But when is it too late to try the diet? Never! *In people whose autistic behaviors are being* caused *by these proteins,* taking away the trigger foods can yield benefits such as reduced anxiety, reduced discomfort, better sleep, better interpersonal contact, and many more improvements:

"Reading your book changed our world. We have dealt with dozens of specialists and experts over the last decade in the quest for an answer as to what was *really* wrong with our daughter. She went on the diet last August and she stopped raging three days later. Stephanie is sixteen, but her (and our!) life has changed dramatically—from a 29 percent scholastic average to a stunning 85 percent this past midterm! I think other parents need to know that it is never too late."

—*Tracey Dynes, Canada*

Recovery is a funny word, anyway. How many of us have quirky relatives who were never diagnosed *with* anything, who are not diagnosable *as* anything but . . . eccentric? How many kids nowadays are "typical"? How many adults are "normal"? Recovery is a "spectrum" in its own right.

The biggest question really isn't "Will my child recover?" After the bleak prognosis of autism, most parents can be grateful for *any* progress that might lead their child to be more comfortable, to learn and grow without intense frustration, or to become a functional member of their family.

For many, a recovery from autism might mean that the child can attend regular school without an aide, or will someday be able to live independently. For some, it merely means he is capable of developing satisfying, reciprocal relationships with family members. For others, it would be a blessed relief if their child would simply sleep through the night, or cease his continuous screaming, or stop hurting himself or others. Regardless of the diagnosis, take pride in your child's achievements as you would any other child's, and think of the recovery process as a journey, not a destination.

Parents often ask whether to put their whole family on the diet. This depends on the child, and the family. If you have a child who will grab food from others' plates, raid the fridge, and climb the pantry shelves to "sniff out" gluten, this might be a good plan.

I know of one little girl whose whole family went on the diet because of her ability to sniff out gluten, and she then began licking the backs of stamps and drinking bottles of wheat-based cosmetics! But this is an extreme case of addiction. For most families, it is not necessary to take such precautions.

I have heard however from many folks that when the whole family went on the diet there were unexpected benefits. For example, Dad's compulsive eating decreased, and he stopped getting "brain fog" after lunch. Meanwhile, Mom was able to stop taking her anxiety medication, and her joint pain all but disappeared; Sis had an easier time paying attention at home and at school, and Little Brother stopped wetting his bed. It is suspected that food allergies, which might result in a range of indistinct symptoms, are common in families with an autistic member, and wheat and milk are common culprits.

Does the gluten- and casein-free diet work for attention deficit disorder (ADD) and other developmental disabilities? Usually not to the degree that we see improvement in some autistic children. However, family members with ADD do often respond noticeably to changes in diet. This is something that we have often heard, and is absolutely worth investigating.

In general, we have heard the most GF/CF success stories associated with children on the autism spectrum. Sometimes these are kids who were not specifically diagnosed with autism or PDD, but have autistic behaviors such as stimming or flapping, or odd social and language skills.

People often want to know how long they need to do the diet. If it is helping, does this mean their child will never eat gluten and casein again? My guess is that for a few kids it may be as simple as allowing time for a "leaky" gut to heal, at which point they might be able to go off the diet.

Some parents have even told me that their child was able to go off the diet after treating an underlying immunological problem, often in the care of doctors or naturopaths using alternative medicine. This is exciting news, and I look forward to hearing further details about such treatments, and more of the long-term results.

However, for many children who have tried to go off the diet after years of success, the reprieve was only temporary, the gut damage recurred, and the behaviors returned in a matter of weeks, often in the form of a more severe psychosis. Perhaps these kids had certain antibodies to gluten, or maybe a pancreatic insufficiency. Autism is a complex disorder, and we just don't fully understand all of the mechanisms which can lead to these behaviors. I always caution parents of diet responders to stick with the diet until we have more answers. It's really not that hard once you get started!

A word of caution: some people will claim that if you give your child certain enzyme formulations, he or she can eat gluten and casein with no ill effects. I have heard from hundreds of parents about this, and it does not appear to be true. It would take only a small amount of casomorphin to flood the opiate receptor sites in the brain, and there is no way to believe that an enzyme tablet can fully break down every peptide that is ingested.

However, digestive enzymes may be helpful in the diet for different reasons. Many other proteins and grains can be problematic, especially if overall digestion is impaired. In addition, keeping a bottle on hand for accidental ingestion of gluten or casein seems to alleviate an adverse reaction. Just remember, it is no substitute for the diet. Why give the antidote along with the poison?

I have another serious concern. Since the first printing of my book, I have heard from many hundreds of parents about the vaccination issue:

"My son Douglas was premature but seemed totally normal until May 25, 1993—MMR day! Within a month he was biting other children."
—*Christie Atkins, Rome, Georgia*

"My son Benjamin (aged two and a half) is autistic, following an assault on his immune system on November 4, 1998 (aged thirteen and a half months). On this day my normally developing son (who said 'Mama,' 'Dada,' 'Sissy,' pointed to objects, and loved to be held) received his diphtheria-tetanus-pertussis, measles-mumps-rubella, Hib, inactivated polio vaccine, and varicella vaccines. He had pinkeye at the time, and had just recovered from an ear infection/upper respiratory infection. I did not know that day what I know now, about the contents of vaccines, the true statistics regarding the risks, and the true nature of some of these 'horrible' diseases I was 'protecting' him from."

—*Catherine Bertrand*

"My two-year-old son, Joey, was diagnosed with MSDD (multisystem developmental disorder) at twenty-three months. He was developing normally until age fifteen months (when he received the MMR). He was talking, giving kisses, playing with everything . . . and then it stopped. He stopped talking, began hand flapping, and was not playing with any of his toys. He was given the shot in August, and by December he had no interest in Christmas or any of his Christmas presents. He just wanted to flap and self-stim."

—*A parent*

The onset of regressive autism in many children coincided with their shots, or with some other immune insult in the first, second, or third year of life. It is my belief that this subtype, once rare, now comprises the majority of cases, and is responsible for the very real increase in the number of young children with autism entering the school systems. The good news is that these kids are usually biologically treatable, and the sooner, the better.

The bad news is that many parents are still not being informed of these treatments until months or years after the diagnosis, and that, despite what our doctors are telling us, we just don't know for sure whether the shots are responsible for triggering autism in some susceptible children. If, indeed, these cases of autism could be prevented, then an immeasurable tragedy is taking place before our eyes.

"My daughter Emma was an excellent baby. She rarely cried, loved to nurse, and smiled at me often. She developed normally, reaching her milestones on time. She played with toys, and interacted with her older sister and with us. At around twelve months she started speaking. She would ask us for juice, or cheese, or milk, cookies, etc. We would tell her to say 'please,' and she would look up at us and smile and say 'PEESE!' We were quite happy with her development.

"When Emma had her MMR shot, she had what would be considered a 'normal' reaction: low-grade fever and sleepiness. Within a short time, we noticed that Emma did not seem to be speaking anymore. We asked each other, 'When was the last time you heard Emma say "Barney"? Or "bath"? "Ball"? "Cookie"?' We sat down one night with paper and pencil and wrote every word we had heard Emma speak—over twenty of them. But all of a sudden she wasn't using them. She wasn't even saying 'Mama' or 'Dada.' We noticed that she seemed not to hear us. She also became extremely constipated.

"She had begun to do 'funny' things. She would take cans out of the food cupboards and line them up, and she would do the same thing with cups, blocks, almost anything. She started spending HOURS flipping the pages back and forth in the phone book, catalogs, even the unabridged dictionary. We noticed that when she saw the credits roll by after a video, she would watch the words, standing on her toes, flapping her hands. She spent incredibly long periods of time in activities that were completely bizarre for a child her age, such as lifting the flap on the pet door and letting it drop. She would do this over and over for so long that we would finally have to physically remove her from the activity, only to have her open and close cabinets for another equally long period of time.

"All of a sudden, we couldn't take Emma anywhere. She would wail and scream and look terrified if we put her in strange surroundings. When she was two and a half, it became obvious that something was just not right. We had tried as best we could to discount her odd behavior, but her distress was getting worse all the time. After a battery of tests, blood work, etc., to rule out other possibilities, Emma was diagnosed with autism in March of 1999. She was nearly three.

"We took Emma to private one-on-one speech and occupational therapy four times a week. We also took her to an additional hour of occupational therapy once a week, and to water/speech therapy once a week. In the fall of 1999, we enrolled her in a special preschool. She was not making progress. She spent most of the time at therapy and school screaming and crying, and was totally uncooperative. Her initial schedule of two days a week at school was too much for her; she was cut back to one day a week, and I had to stay with her the whole time. She could not even sit in a chair, let alone complete a task. In March of 2000 (two months ago), we read your book, cleaned out the cupboards, and started the GF/CF diet within three days.

"Within the last two months, Emma has improved dramatically. Her eye contact is nearly normal. She has done so well at preschool that we now drop her off at the door to the classroom, and she walks right in. We have increased her to four days a week. She no longer stays up until 4 or 5 A.M. She now goes to sleep at eight, and sleeps soundly until seven in the morning. She is no longer constipated.

"We have been able to take her off of imipramine, the antidepressant she started taking when she started hitting her head on the floor. She no longer needs it; she is happier than we have ever seen her. She transitions well, she responds to her name, and last week she said 'My dad!' when she saw my husband. Today she played ring-around-the-rosy with her sisters. She held a doll two days ago and pretended to nurse it. Everyone who knows her is in awe of the changes, including her doctor.

"I apologize for the length of this letter, as I know you are busy. You have changed our lives, and for that I will be eternally grateful. I saw absolutely no autistic behaviors in Emma before the MMR. She steadily worsened until we implemented this diet, which has been our greatest blessing.

"Thank you so much! If I can do *anything* to raise awareness of autism, I will gladly do it. I am more than happy to share my story, especially if it will help someone else. I used to lie awake at night wondering if I would ever hear my daughter say, 'I love you,' and if I can spare even one parent that pain, I will have accomplished a miracle."

—*Jaymee R. Dever, Lewiston, Idaho*

The above letter is a classic example of the many children, like my son, who regressed and then responded to dietary intervention.

Children with regressive autism, insensitivity to pain, GI symptoms, self-limited ("picky") diets, and sleep problems are *almost
always* diet responders. However, those with *none* of the above
symptoms may also improve on the diet. The only way to know for
certain (since urine testing is not terribly accurate) is to *try the diet.*
Do it right, and do it for at least three months. Think you can't?
Think again!

Top 10 Reasons Why People Say They Don't Want to Try the Diet
  10. It sounds too hard.
   9. I don't know how to cook.
   8. My doctor doesn't believe in it (or: I'm a doctor and I know
       better).
   7. His other parent (or teachers, grandparents, etc.) won't go
       along with it.
   6. We believe behavioral therapy will recover him.
   5. I'm afraid it won't work.
   4. I'm afraid it WILL work.
   3. I don't want to take away his favorite foods, because Food =
       Love.
   2. I'm worried about his nutrition—even though he presently
       eats only Cheerios and Cheez Doodles.

and . . .

   1. He'll *starve* if I take away milk and wheat.

These last two are the worst reasons of all—many kids with this
opiate problem self-limit to these foods, and so are among the most
likely to respond to the diet!

If you've tried the diet and your child is a diet responder, you have
great reason to be hopeful. If your child has a different subtype of au-

tism, it is up to you to look for his or her "magic bullet"—don't wait for the medical community to do it for you! I believe the answers are out there, and that someday every form of autism will be found to be treatable. But I also believe it is the parents of these children who will lead us to the answers.

—Karyn Seroussi, December 2001

PART ONE

Miles's Story:

Hunting the Jabberwock

Prologue

We're in the emergency room. It's three o'clock in the morning and Miles has been screaming for two hours. His limbs are tremoring. Are these seizures? They started before his fever went up. His temperature is 106 degrees. Could this be related to his eighteen-month DPT (diphtheria, pertussis, tetanus) vaccination the previous morning? The doctor doesn't know. The same thing happened three months ago, a few days after his MMR (measles, mumps, rubella) vaccination. Now his fever is breaking and he is lying limply in my arms. He is staring into my eyes with a surprised look. He smiles slightly. I have a sudden feeling of elation. "It's me, it's Mommy," I whisper. He stares for several minutes, as if memorizing my face. I relish his gaze. I'll never forget this moment. It is the first time in three months he has let me look into those beautiful eyes. It will not happen again for a long, long time.

Miles resisted my efforts to hold him and climbed off my lap. He toddled over to the microphone and tried to pull it off its Formica table. It was screwed down, so he contented himself with swiveling it from side to side. I looked up at the one-way glass. Were we being observed?

I really didn't think so. Perhaps the evaluation was being videotaped. I decided that I should be interacting with Miles, just in case.

"Milo, come here, sweetie." He ignored me, so I went over to him and pulled him away from the microphone. I sat him on my lap, facing me, and tried to charm him into a game of patty-cake. He whined and bent over sideways, straining to get away. I put his hands in front of his face, then took them away.

"Where's Milo? Peekaboo!" His whining grew louder and more high-pitched. "Where's Milo?"

That question stayed in my head as I let him go. He went back to the microphone as I bit my lip. I realized, for the first time, how Miles's behavior must appear to others. Didn't all nineteen-month-olds love to play peekaboo? Didn't he once love games like that? What was wrong with him?

I had been warned not to compare my children, but my daughter, Laura, had adored the times we set aside to sing songs, tumble on the floor, and play lap games. At nineteen months she would climb into my bed each morning for at least half an hour, smiling into my eyes and making me teach her words.

"What dat?"

"That's a pillow."

"Piw-low. What dat?"

"That's a ceiling fan."

"Seewing fan."

Miles wanted little to do with us, and showed no interest in our language. Sometimes he ran to me when he was injured, his face contorted with misery, running almost into my arms and then turning, suddenly, so that I had to pick him up from behind.

He had said a few words as early as eleven months old: "cat," "Mama-ma-ma," "dance," "yay!" But that was months ago. There was "ish," his word for "fish," which had also disappeared.

The door opened. Beth and Bonnie sat down at the little table with the colored cubes still stacked into tiny towers. The room was very warm, and I looked out the window into the parking lot. A breeze blew the trees outside. Did these windows open? Probably not. Rooms with one-way glass are not likely to have windows that open.

Beth was speaking. The room, the table, and the whole scene had become slightly unreal, as if I were watching myself act in a play.

"We've analyzed Miles's test scores. He does have some irregularities in his development. Motor skills are a relative strength, but his language is severely delayed."

On the back of a large white envelope, Beth began writing numbers for me to look at. Numbers that meant Miles was developmentally delayed. My skin began to crawl.

"Miles's language development is at less than a six-month level, and his social skills are at about ten months."

But Miles was nineteen months old. How could something be so seriously amiss without anyone having noticed? He had passed his twelve-month and fifteen-month checkups with flying colors.

"We think that Miles has a disorder somewhere along the autistic spectrum."

"Autistic?" I whispered. "Do you mean autism?"

"We now refer to it as the 'autistic spectrum.' He could be on the very mild end, and he's so young, it's hard to know for sure. It's a developmental disorder, accounting for a range of delays including language and social development."

What did that mean? She didn't make it sound too bad. I stared at Miles, a tall, handsome little boy with a sturdy body, fair curls, and rosy cheeks. He looked normal. Strangely enough, I was reassured. In a way, it was good to know that what was wrong had a name. I felt a glimmer of relief that someone had finally acknowledged my concerns. But autism? The word conjured up a vague image of a profoundly disturbed child rocking in a corner. Suddenly, I felt a surge of adrenaline and my heart began to pound.

Miles finally left the swiveling microphone, crossed the room, and began to open and close the door of a toy barn on the table. First he opened it, took the cow out, and closed it, then opened it, put the cow back, and closed it again.

"Does he do a lot of repetitive things like that at home?" asked Bonnie Kramer, a psychologist.

"Well, he has a scientific mind, like his father. Alan is a research chemist. Miles likes to systematically experiment with a toy like that. I don't think of it as repetitive, really. I mean, since he varies it. See? This time he took out the farmer and the cow." I paused. "It's very hot in here, isn't it?"

They were silent.

"What does this mean?"

"Well, we're going to refer you to a developmental pediatrician for a formal diagnosis," Beth said. "But right now we're going to have you speak with our social worker. I'll play with Miles for a while until you're done."

"I don't think he'll let me leave him with strangers," I said.

I was wrong.

CHAPTER ONE

The Diagnosis

A severe language delay is almost never diagnosed in a child under two, and autism is tricky—sometimes there are a few words and normal developmental milestones in the beginning and it's hard to notice when they disappear or don't increase. Besides, so many well-meaning people had reassured me:

> You can't compare him to Laura—she was so precocious.
> Boys talk later than girls do.
> He's had so many ear infections.
> Alan didn't talk until he was three.
> My next-door neighbor's son didn't talk until he was four.
> Einstein didn't talk until he was . . .

I had changed pediatricians twice, begging for help or information regarding Miles's irregular sleep patterns and chronic ear infections. At that time, when he was a year old, his social development was not yet a problem, but his ears were. The first two doctors had concurred in a misdiagnosis of asthma due to his mucusy breathing, and prescribed

albuterol, a medication that opens bronchial tubes, in the words of the
first doctor, "to use if the noise bothers you."

"My mother just read an article linking milk and wheat to ear
infections," I had explained to the second doctor. "Do you think I
should try taking him off those foods?"

"The medical community doesn't put much stock in those studies," she had said. "You can try it if you like."

"Well, Miles loves milk. I'd hate to take it away if I don't have to."

"It probably won't make a difference anyway. Some kids just get ear
infections. They'll clear up in the spring."

I had doubted that the ear infections would "clear up" by themselves. Alan and I had had the same disconcerting feeling that we
would never again sleep through the night.

After eight ear infections in three months, and countless doses of
antibiotics, I had asked the doctor if she would recommend ear tubes
for Miles.

"I don't like medicating him so often," I had explained. "It seems
like he's always on antibiotics. And he's up for so much of the night.
I am really not functioning very well on so little sleep, and Laura is
finding his constant crying extremely stressful."

"Well, some children require more effort than others. Just because
you had an easy time with Laura doesn't mean there's something wrong
with Miles."

"Yes, I realize that, but he is just *so* difficult. I own a retail business,
and I can't tell you how many times I've had to leave work to bring
him in. And the screaming . . . I'm sure there's something wrong with
him. I thought that if he had ear tubes . . ."

The doctor had looked at me coldly.

"Parenting can sometimes interfere with our work schedules," she
had said. "Perhaps you are the one who needs help, not Miles."

I was stunned. I had stared at her for a moment, then turned
around and walked out of that office for the last time.

This event begins our story. I was to learn that the next chapter of our lives was not to be unique. To other parents of autistic children, it was a hauntingly familiar sequence of events.

Dr. Stover, our new pediatrician, was booked up when we switched to her practice, so on January 12 we saw her nurse-practitioner, Susan Percy.

"What about his breathing?" I asked. "We were told it was asthma, but the albuterol doesn't seem to make a difference. Can you hear it? It's not really wheezing. It's sort of a honking or clucking in the back of his throat."

Mrs. Percy listened for a moment. Then she went out and came back with Dr. Stover, who smiled and introduced herself. Miles picked up his shirt from the examining table and used it to play peekaboo with her while she put a stethoscope to his chest.

"Cute baby," she said, smiling. "Who told you that was asthma?"

"Two different doctors. What is it?"

"Just mucus," she said. "I don't know what causes that—allergies maybe—but don't worry about it. When he's old enough to clear his throat, it will go away. You can throw away the albuterol—it won't help."

"I didn't think it did," I said, smiling with relief.

In mid-February I was back in her office. I explained that I was concerned because Miles's language development seemed slower than Laura's had been.

"From what you've told me, Laura was an early talker," said Dr. Stover. "At this age, at thirteen months or so, two or three words is perfectly normal. Miles's social development looks good—I wouldn't worry. But I will send you over to Otolaryngology for a hearing test. I agree that he has had an awful lot of ear infections."

Two weeks later, on March 3, Miles did fairly well on the test. He showed only a very mild hearing loss—"within normal parameters."

We visited the office again a month later, on April 4, for Miles's fifteen-month well-baby visit.

"Miles's ears look good."

"Yes, well, they should. Alan says we should buy stock in amoxicillin. But one more ear infection and he's getting ear tubes—Dr. Roberts at Oto gave me his solemn promise."

Ear infections occur when fluid builds up in the inner ear. "Tubes," which are called "grommets" in England, are little rubber cylinders that are installed in the eardrum to help alleviate the pressure and hopefully prevent further infections. While the child is anesthetized, his doctor makes a tiny incision in the eardrum and inserts the tube as if it were a window between two rooms.

Mrs. Percy laughed and handed me a form to sign, authorizing them to give Miles his measles-mumps-rubella vaccine.

"What happens if I don't sign this?" I asked.

"Well, you won't be able to send Miles to nursery school, or kindergarten."

"Oh. Okay. It's just that these risk warnings are kind of scary."

"Well, vaccine reactions are very rare. Try not to think about it."

"Okay. But first, can you give him some Tylenol? He had a really bad screaming episode after his two-month DPT shot."

Three days later I was back. Miles had another ear infection.

Eight days after the shot, on April 12, after giving me another lecture about how the medical community was trying to be more conservative about inserting ear tubes, the otolaryngologist approved the surgery. It would be at the end of the month, just before our trip to Los Angeles to visit Alan's family.

Then, two days after that, Miles had a really miserable day. It was the first night of Passover, a night when my family always came together from different parts of the country. I was having the Seder, the ceremonial dinner, at my house, and was frantically trying to prepare. Fortunately, I had arranged for Lyn, our baby-sitter, to stay for dinner and to put the children to bed. Miles was pale and cranky, and barely acknowledged his grandmother or his adored Uncle Matthew. He cried during the meal and refused to eat, instead drinking several cups of milk. Lyn put him to bed early.

Late that night, only an hour after I finished cleaning the kitchen, Miles was up screaming. His face was red and his limbs seemed to be shaking. Alan put some liquid ibuprofen in a cup with a couple of ounces of milk, but no sooner did Miles drink it than he threw up. Over the screaming I hollered to Alan to find the thermometer— Miles was beginning to feel warm.

By the time Alan found the thermometer Miles was very, very hot. I measured his temperature at 106. His limbs were trembling violently, and his screams had intensified. I threw him into his car seat and drove the two miles to the hospital as fast as I could, running two red lights in the quiet streets.

Finally, after three Tylenol suppositories, Miles stopped crying and fell asleep. The resident at the emergency room did not have an explanation.

The next three weeks were strange ones. Miles seemed very spaced out. He stopped talking, stopped smiling, and started drinking a lot of milk.

Then, at exactly sixteen months old, Miles got his ear tubes. In the waiting room, before the surgery, he held my hand as we watched the tropical fish swim peacefully in a large tank. "Ishhhhh," he whispered, for the last time.

After the surgery the doctor told us he had had something called "glue ear."

"The fluid in his ear had hardened into a thick gum, like Silly Putty," he said. "It must have been causing a bit of discomfort and perhaps some mild hearing loss."

"What causes that? Could that be from allergies? My mother thinks ear infections are caused by milk allergy."

"I don't know about that. I do see this in some children. It's good that we got in there, since masses like that harbor infection and take a long time to go away by themselves. You're probably going to see a real explosion in his language now."

"Thank you so much," I said, relieved. "We're so glad to have this over with." Alan picked up our dazed son and carried him out to the car.

"Now maybe things will get back to normal," he said.

But things did not.

Soon we forgot what normal was.

My father-in-law was very ill, and we knew that it was the last time our children would ever see him. I brought the video camera on our trip to California, and taped much of our visit. Laura was so cute, singing songs and telling stories in her squeaky little voice, golden ringlets bouncing around her head.

Meanwhile, in the background, Miles trotted back and forth across a patch of gravel in his grandparents' backyard. Back and forth, back and forth. Several times I tried to engage him, my voice on the videotape sounding cheerful but with an obvious note of concern.

"Hi, Miles! Hi, sweetie! Whatcha doing?"

Miles would turn and stare at the camera, unsmiling, for a few seconds, then turn away. There was no joy, no sadness, no curiosity, no connection, nothing. I moved the camera away from my face and tried again.

"Miles! Miles! Milo! Miles!"

He finally turned and looked at me as if I were a few lines of incomprehensible hieroglyphics, a meaningless combination of features. Chilled, I turned off the camera.

At the table that evening, in his high chair, I saw a faint glimmer of acknowledgment as he recognized a familiar command. "Milo, make bang-bang! Make bang-bang!" I smacked both hands on the table to show him. He knew this; he had done this before. It was one of his favorite games. I felt a twinge of fear. Suddenly, he responded, just for a moment, patting the table with his hands. Then, abruptly, he looked away. I could not get him to do it again.

After our trip, life became much worse. Miles's stools had become very loose, with a sour, pungent smell, and he became more and more withdrawn.

One day I was trying to get lunch ready before Miles woke up. Please, just one more minute. He could read my mind. I heard a whine from the baby monitor on the kitchen windowsill. I had forgotten to make a bottle. Urgently, I rinsed off my hands and poured milk into a bottle, screwing on the nipple as I ran upstairs. Sometimes, if he got the bottle fast enough . . . but it was too late. The whines had turned to screams.

Every time he woke up, every morning and after every nap, Miles would cry inconsolably for about half an hour. Nothing seemed to help, and nothing distracted him. I could tell that Lyn, our baby-sitter, was close to quitting.

"Babies are not supposed to cry this much," she said over the din, as if I had some control over the duration of his screaming.

I looked at her helplessly. Aren't some babies just high-strung?

"Miles, cut it out! Stop!" Alan once shouted. He so rarely raised his voice to the children; it actually startled Miles into stopping, for a moment. Then he began to scream again.

"Miles, Miles, you're giving me a migraine," Alan said.

"Maybe *he's* got a migraine," I suggested. "Look at how he's rubbing his forehead on your chest." I took over for a while, holding him and making soothing noises, for my own comfort, I suppose, since it seemed to make little difference to the unhappy child in my arms.

Sometimes, after ten or fifteen minutes, we could get him to stop with a bottle of milk and a Disney sing-along video. I remember the feeling of relief when the moving images finally caught his attention and the screaming began to ease up. I would hold perfectly still with him in my arms, afraid to move. After a few minutes, my muscles would begin to ache, and I would ease him onto the couch, moving so slowly and noiselessly that even my cat wouldn't have noticed.

After a while, we found ourselves relying on those videos a lot.

"Hey, Alan, remember before we had kids, when we agreed that we disapproved of TV for young children?"

Alan just looked at me grimly.

We got into the habit of keeping cups of milk handy at all times, just to avoid the screaming. On ice, in our bedroom, for at least one nighttime awakening. Three cups in the diaper bag for a two-hour trip to the mall.

I was at my store. A frequent customer of mine, Patty, was there with her little boy. Her son was the same age as mine and was also not really talking, although he said a couple of words. I smiled at him. He smiled back. Patty prompted him.

"Jimmy, can you say hi to Karyn?" His grin widened. "He's started saying hi," she explained. Suddenly, he pointed at a poster behind me, which had a picture of a bird on it.

"Look!" he said excitedly.

At that very moment my mind became firmly unsettled. My belief that my children were safe and healthy was seriously threatened for the very first time since I had become a parent. At first I couldn't put my finger on it, but there was something about what Patty's son had just done that mine simply could not do. Then I realized that he had *pointed*.

Just what was it about pointing that was so special? I recognized that it was a child's request for shared attention, his way of saying "I want you to see what I'm seeing." Miles did not seem to care about things like that. When Laura was a toddler, I could hardly sit down before she filled my lap with items to share with me, or for me to appreciate with her. She had pointed regularly, while Miles did not. What I didn't realize at the time was that the absence of pointing is one of the defining characteristics of autism.

I made another appointment with the pediatrician. Lyn arrived at my house fifteen minutes late to watch Laura. I found myself in a panic.

"I'm sorry," Lyn said breathlessly, "I had to drop my puppy off at the vet."

Seething, I grabbed Miles and flew out to the car. Usually calm about being late, I was in a frenzy. When the receptionist told me we'd have to reschedule, I started to cry.

"I have to see her," I said.

"I'm sorry, but this was scheduled as a nonurgent visit, and you are fifteen minutes late," she said.

"It is urgent," I lied. "Miles woke up this morning with a very bad cough."

"Hold on, let me check."

While she phoned back to the nurse, I wiped my eyes and realized with some surprise how anxious I really was about my son. I had barely let myself think about this appointment until it was in jeopardy of being canceled. Now I knew I had to have some answers.

"The nurse-practitioner can see you, if you like."

"Great. That's great. Thank you."

I liked Susan Percy. She was a patient and thoughtful woman, and I was sure she would listen. She smiled as she pulled out her clipboard.

"So, tell me about Miles's cough."

"Um, he doesn't have a cough. But I really needed to see you."

She nodded and leaned against the door. I tried to put my uneasiness into words.

"Miles doesn't seem to understand anything we say. Not even the word 'cup,' which is his favorite thing in the world. The other day I held the cup behind my back and said, 'Want your cup? Cup?' There was no reaction until he actually *saw* the cup, and then he went nuts. I know some kids talk late, but don't they usually have *some* understanding of language? My brother's son Teddy is about the same age and he doesn't talk much, but if I say 'Give this to Daddy,' he'll run and do it."

She hesitated for a moment, but did not look alarmed. She looked over at Miles, who was opening and closing a drawer under the examining table. "Miles! Miles? Miles!" She spoke sharply. The third time she said his name, Miles looked around vaguely and then went back to his business of playing with the drawer. Open, close. She shrugged slightly.

"He should have some receptive language by now, that's true. His hearing seems to be okay . . . Otolaryngology didn't find anything. Let's send him over to Hearing and Speech, and find out what they have to say. Just to see what's going on."

I was relieved, although I don't know what I thought I would hear. Certainly not the word "autism." But at least now my concerns would be taken seriously.

I'm waiting for my sister in a bookstore. What if they have a book about autism? Would it sound familiar? Would it account for my son's peculiarities? Miles does like to be held sometimes, but only on his terms. As a baby, he never loved being rocked, cuddled, or sung to, but he was very loving and responsive. He did say "cat" and "fish," even though he hasn't said them in months. Does he love watching his sister play? How long has it been since I've seen him watching her? Alan was slow. But Bonnie said that speech delay is common in the parents of children with autism. Here it is: the Child Development section. Let's see—Barry Kaufman, some guy with a beard writing about loving a child back from autism. If this were about love, Miles wouldn't have a problem. What else is there? A Parent's Guide to Autism. That sounds useful. Not that Miles has it. After all, he's only had a preliminary diagnosis. But it couldn't hurt to buy the book.

In *A Parent's Guide to Autism,* Charles Hart described abnormal language such as echolalia (repeating another person's words or phrases); bizarre movements, including twirling and hand flapping; and complete lack of awareness of others. It sounded awful, and every therapy used to treat autism involved simply managing the abnormal behaviors. It didn't sound much like Miles, but then again it was supposed to be describing older individuals.

However, the book did describe something called "perseverative play," which sounded uncomfortably familiar. We had a Sit 'n Spin toy at home that Miles liked to take apart by pulling out the stem and replacing it, over and over. He once did that for twenty minutes. And once, in the sandbox, he poured a cup of sand over and over for forty-five minutes. I had referred to this as a long attention span.

Muriel, my mother-in-law, reminded me that Alan had also done things like that. Every time I had had an anxious feeling about Miles, the same reassuring thoughts would appear. For years I had heard from Muriel how different Alan had been as a baby. How late he had begun talking, and then in full sentences.

So many times I had listened to the story about how Alan had figured out how to make a pipe bomb at the age of eight, using household ingredients. He was discovered when he tried to blow up an ant-hill and took out half of the sidewalk in front of his aunt's house. It was a classic family anecdote—the punch line was that Alan ended up with a Ph.D. in chemistry.

Alan had memorized the encyclopedia by the age of eleven, and still remembered all of it. He could tell you the structural difference between a piano and a harpsichord, or between a grasshopper and a locust. He knew the electronic properties of tourmaline, the exact path of the Gulf Stream, the diameter of the moon, and the names and dates of all of the monarchs of England.

After a while I took this for granted. The late language, the superb memory, the perfect pitch, the dyslexia, and even the mildly erratic social skills—these were all part of what made Alan fascinating and unique. Of course, he had often been compared to Albert Einstein, who was reputed to have similar traits along with his brilliant mind.

Shortly after we met, I brought Alan to a party at my sister's house. I overheard a stranger ask him what he did. Alan began to describe the specific DNA project that he was working on at the time, much to the obvious confusion of the listener. I jumped in with, "Alan is a research chemist. He's doing a postdoc at Columbia." Later I chided him about it. "Start with the general, then move to the specific."

"He asked what kind of work I do."

"Alan, how did you get to be thirty without knowing what that question means? It means 'What is your profession?'"

"Oh."

"Remember that time we played Pictionary with Cathy and Bob? Your clue was something like 'door handle' and you just drew a line and kept pointing to it. You have to draw the door first, to put it in context for other people."

"Got it."

For a while, I tried to become Alan's social tutor. Listening to him speak with others, I always knew when a misunderstanding was about to strike. I began to predict how Alan would interpret something that he heard, and to jump in and elucidate. I grew accustomed to seeing the perplexed look on someone's face and intervening with an explanation.

"Okay, okay," Alan would say patiently, after I explained my interference. "I understand." He did, too. Once corrected, he rarely made the same type of mistake again. But how odd that he didn't know these things intuitively.

After we were married, I learned to stop. I realized that Alan did make himself understood quite well, just in a different way than I would have. In fact, he was rather perceptive in ways in which I was not, and his instincts for judging character were unusually good.

Anyway, Alan was so smart, and so handsome, that such awkward moments usually passed unnoticed. I was pleased to have found such a fascinating and intelligent husband. And he *was* fascinating. I had never before met a man who was so utterly intriguing. He could answer all of my questions about nature, science, history, weather, archaeology . . . and yet he was so helpless when it came to simple matters like putting away groceries.

My mother once laughed and assured me that this was true of other men, but she didn't understand the real differences that I saw in my husband. He was just on a different plane. A higher one, perhaps, but one that left him slightly detached from the real world. *Or, at least, the world that I thought was the "real" one.*

Although I teased him about his grasp of social protocol, I had to admit that Alan was a deeply passionate person. He just had such a different view of things. When we met, he thought that every bus driver was a poet. He had no idea, until I told him, that most people saw things differently than he did.

On the night he proposed, Alan took my hand and stood with me under the stars, outside a restaurant in Connecticut. "I can teach you all about the world," he said, "and you can teach me how to live in it."

He did, and I did. And our marriage has been a good one.

Now I was beginning to see that Alan, and possibly other "eccentric geniuses" of our time, might lie somewhere in the gray area that lay between what Beth had called the autistic spectrum and the rest of humanity. But Miles was much worse than Alan ever was. Alan was highly intelligent, and, according to his parents, he had been language-delayed, but he was *not* autistic. What had caused the difference?

I continued to read *A Parent's Guide to Autism.* It didn't say anything about diagnosing autism in babies, but it did mention something intriguing: a book called *Fighting for Tony,* by Mary Callahan. Her little boy had been misdiagnosed with autism when what he really had was a rare "cerebral allergy" to milk. A cerebral allergy? I was skeptical. I knew something about biology, and I'd never heard that food allergies could make your brain swell, without other classic allergic symptoms. But milk? Apparently, Tony had recovered from autism when he was taken off milk. The chances of that seemed pretty slim, but then I remembered something else Muriel had said about Alan's childhood.

"When Alan was three, he was a fat baby—what they used to call a 'milk baby.' Oh, he loved his milk. He wasn't walking, probably because he was so fat, and he didn't talk. He didn't need to, of course. All he had to do was grunt, and his big sister would bring him whatever he wanted.

"Anyway, my cousin Florence, a psychiatrist, came over for a visit and told me that Alan was mentally retarded. I was terribly upset. I rushed him to our doctor, Dr. Miller, but he was only concerned that Alan was drinking so much milk, since the only other thing he ate was applesauce. Dr. Miller said that Alan was anemic, and that we had to take milk out of his diet so that he would eat other foods. Then Alan was much better, and he started walking and talking soon after."

What else had I heard about milk? Oh yes. Bonnie Kramer, the psychologist from Hearing and Speech, had told me that her daughter had screamed like Miles as a baby, but stopped when they took dairy products out of her diet. And then there was that article my mother had shown me about ear infections and dairy or wheat allergies.

I decided to get *Fighting for Tony* from the library. Alan had gone to the library the week before, but all he would say about what he found out was that the best educational program for Miles was something he called "Lovaas."

He was terribly anxious. We were both consumed with worry, but Alan handled stress especially badly. Every morning he would wake up the same way: snap off the alarm clock and wordlessly take a shower. Then, as he dressed, he would ask me to retell the story of what Beth had said at the appointment. "But what were her exact words? Did she say he was profoundly autistic?"

"No, I told you she didn't. She said he *might* be on the autistic spectrum."

"But that he's mentally retarded."

"No, Alan, she did *not* say he was mentally retarded. She said there did not appear to be mental retardation. The book said that mental retardation is associated with autism. That's probably because nonverbal children score very low on IQ tests."

"But she was sure that he has autism?"

"No, that's what this Dr. Hyman will tell us. Why do you keep asking me this over and over?"

Distressed, I would get into the shower myself. Alan would go to work without saying good-bye.

One morning, as I pulled the cotton out of a new bottle of aspirin, I watched, transfixed, as the fibers stretched and began to separate. I stared at the pieces, strained to the point of breaking, held tenuously between my fingers. One more centimeter and they would completely come apart. This was my marriage, my family, my life.

I called my doctor and asked for a referral to a crisis counselor. Then I went to the library. I sat in front of the library computer and began the word search. *Two entries matching autism.* It was August 1995, and there were only two books on autism at my local branch. I also found a chapter in a 1980 book about developmental delays, which sounded pretty much like the *Parent's Guide.* Its conclusion was: Prognosis—Poor. Again, there wasn't much written about what autism looks like in babies, and that's what I desperately wanted to know.

I pulled the two books from the shelves. One was called *Russell Is Extra Special,* by Dr. Charles Amenta III. It was a beautiful photographic children's book about a little boy named Russell who lived in a world of his own in the midst of a loving family. With each turn of the page I could feel my heart breaking. "Russell likes to eat with his fingers," the book explained. Looking at the picture of Russell in the bathtub with his brothers, I could feel the fear rising in my throat. His

brothers were smiling at the camera. Sandwiched between them physically, Russell smiled, too, but he was clearly in another place. Unaware
of their very existence, right there in the same bathtub.

Chilled, I pushed away the feeling of panic. This will not happen
to Miles, I vowed. I had always dealt with frightening situations by
taking control of them, but if Miles really had autism it seemed that I
was helpless. Russell's father was a doctor. There was nothing he could
do but tell his son's story.

I looked at the second book, *Let Me Hear Your Voice,* by Catherine
Maurice, which appeared more promising. It was described as the tri-
umphant story of two children who had fully recovered from autism.
Okay, so there may be something I can do. I decided to wait until after
Miles's formal diagnosis to read that one.

Before I left the library, almost as an afterthought, I grabbed a
copy of *Is This Your Child?* by Doris Rapp. It was about how allergies
could have behavioral as well as physical manifestations. It sounded
far-fetched, but I was hoping it might say something about "cerebral
allergies."

> *If this is so common, why haven't I heard of it before? I just discovered*
> *that there are two other children with autism on my street. Why wasn't*
> *I warned? This is not happening to me. I didn't sign up for this. I'm*
> *not cut out to be one of those noble parents of the disabled. But what*
> *if it is true? What if my beautiful, perfect baby has a severe, lifelong*
> *disability? The answer is this pain in my body. The answer is that my*
> *child has been kidnapped and no officials can be notified, no suspects*
> *can be questioned. Life goes on as usual, but my baby's soul and spirit*
> *are gone.*

The Doris Rapp book was fascinating, although I could see that it
lacked the criteria for traditional scientific credibility. A skeptic married to a scientist, at that time I took lightly her reports of miraculous

recoveries from ADD (attention deficit disorder) by dietary changes. I couldn't find anything about "cerebral allergies." But I did find something interesting: according to Dr. Rapp, an individual with a milk allergy is likely to suffer from ear infections, irritability, poor sleeping habits, and a craving for the very food to which he is allergic.

I felt a spark of hope. We would take Miles off milk and dairy. Although Miles's diarrhea hadn't started until recently, I was lactose intolerant and it *was* possible that Miles had the same problem digesting milk sugar. At the very least it might stop his diarrhea. And even if it just helped him to sleep better, it was worth a try.

"Alan started talking when we took him off milk," Muriel reminded me on the phone from California. "Maybe Miles is anemic."

"Sure, maybe he is," I said, sighing. If only it were that simple.

Later, I asked Alan about it. "Tell me again what your parents said about you as a baby."

"Well, I didn't speak before my third birthday. Supposedly, I just grunted when I wanted something, or pulled my mother's hand. I drank lots of milk, ate lots of applesauce, and spent my time sitting quietly in my crib, turning a toy over and over, or lining up my Matchbox cars across a doorway."

"Yikes. I know I have heard this many times from your mother, but I didn't know what to make of it. I guess I had disregarded the tale as probable fiction. Now it takes on so much meaning."

But when I questioned Muriel further, I grew more confused.

"Well, sure, he did things like that, but he was really social. He wasn't autistic, he was always smiling. He was a wonderful baby."

So why hadn't Alan gotten worse?

"Muriel, did Alan ever get ear infections as a baby?"

"Well, he was rarely sick, which might be because the climate here in California is so mild."

"So you don't remember giving him antibiotics for any ear infections?"

"Hmm. When he was fussy, and seemed like he had an earache,

I *never* rushed him off to the doctor, and anyway, in those days the doctor didn't just push antibiotics at you to make you go away. I think I remember the doctor giving Alan eardrops, but not oral antibiotics. We'd use warm olive oil on a cotton ball, put it in the ear, and wait it out for a couple of days."

"Did he get them after you took away milk?"

"No, I don't think so."

As an afterthought, I remembered something I had read that linked autism to immunizations.

"What about vaccines? Did he get his shots?"

"Yes, but mostly when he was much older. We didn't give them to babies. He was almost two when he had his first DPT, and three when he got the polio vaccine. He didn't get the measles vaccine until he was about five."

"I actually remember getting the MMR for the first time," I mused. "It was in 1977. I was twelve."

In fact, I had had the MMR more than once. For some reason I never held a titer to rubella, and, as a result, in the past fifteen years I had been revaccinated four more times. I wasn't sure why they didn't just give me the rubella shot alone. Presumably that would have meant a special order.

I thought about the last time I had the MMR and startled myself with the recollection. Miles had been four hours old. I was in the hospital after the delivery and a nurse came in with a syringe in her hand.

"I'm breastfeeding," I told her. "Will the vaccine affect the baby?"

She hesitated. "We do this all the time. It's standard procedure. If you contract rubella during a future pregnancy it can be very serious, so this will protect you."

"Why do you think I never hold a titer to the disease?" I asked, signing the consent form.

"You probably got a bad batch of the vaccine," she replied.

"A bad batch? Four times? Wow. That's not very comforting. Maybe it's just something about my immune system?" I settled back in bed and waited for the sting of the needle. I was too tired to think about it. But from time to time since then the memory has flitted back to me and made me wonder.

Taking away milk and dairy seemed easy enough. We decided to give it a try. Surprisingly, Miles handled the switch back to soy formula very well. He still refused water and drank quite a bit of the formula, but not as much as the milk. We discovered rice milk, which had an odd, sweet taste, and which Miles also accepted.

I have always preferred action to prayer when I have problems to solve. However, I put out a silent all-points bulletin to whatever external powers might control the destinies of helpless little children and begged, please, let Miles be like Tony Callahan and let his autism be a misdiagnosis.

One week later my spark of hope had grown to a flickering flame. Although his stools were still loose, Miles was not screaming nearly as much and was sleeping through the night. Three weeks later his eye contact was much better. We could really see a difference. And he actually took my hand and pulled me to the stairs when he wanted to go down and eat breakfast.

Dr. Susan Hyman was a serious, gentle person with wonderfully kind eyes. She was one of the best developmental pediatricians at one of the best university hospitals in the country. She spent a long time talking to us and examining Miles, listening carefully to our theories, opinions, and questions.

"What about the fact that we took him off the milk?" Alan asked. "Could that be helping? I didn't start talking until my parents took me off milk. The day we switched him to soy, his sleeping started to get better, and his screaming isn't nearly as bad."

"There was this little boy who was misdiagnosed with autism because of a milk allergy," I added.

"I think that's very interesting." She sounded sincere, but I detected a hint of pity in her voice. She could see that we were putting too much hope into the allergy/misdiagnosis theory. "And if you think it seems to be helping, then it can't do any harm. Kids don't really need to drink milk. Make sure he gets enough calcium."

"Does Miles have autism?" Alan asked.

"Well, autism is diagnosed based on certain behavioral criteria. They are pretty specific, and quite obvious to someone who is familiar with them. I'm afraid Miles meets these criteria, and that yes, he does have autism."

Alan didn't move. His face was frozen. Then he spoke softly.

"Is it mild, moderate, or severe?"

"Well," she said, looking at us a bit anxiously, "I'd say moderate. But he's very young, and I have no doubt that the quality of the intervention that you two provide will make a big difference. From what I've heard, he has already improved since he was seen at Hearing and Speech. Focused, one-on-one play is very good for these kids."

CHAPTER TWO

A Plan of Action

FLASHBACKS

There had been a time in my youth when the altering of the mind's perceptions was considered by most young people to be a fascinating diversion. Experimentation with recreational drugs had been one of the great mistakes of my generation, but at least something useful had come from it: I was able to recognize the signs of a chemically altered mind.

Alan was getting ready to leave for work.

"Alan, do you remember that time, a long time ago, when I told you about taking those mushrooms?"

"Yes."

"I was just wondering if you remember saying that it sounded like what your childhood felt like—with intense colors, heightened sensory experiences, a fascination with certain objects, difficulty relating to others . . ."

"Sure. Wasn't yours?"

"No, not mine. I never experienced anything even remotely like it."

"Well, that's the way the world seemed to me when I was little. I remember it all in vivid detail. Can we discuss this later?"

I went downstairs in my pajamas and rooted through my filing cabinet. Impatiently, I pulled out some information about autism that the speech pathologist from Hearing and Speech had sent me. Included was an excellent paper written by Dr. Stephen Bauer, a developmental pediatrician who worked at a local hospital. I sat down to write him a letter.

September 16, 1995

Dear Dr. Bauer:

As the mother of a twenty-month-old recently diagnosed with autistic disorder, I would like to share with you some unusual insight that I have about autism.

I know you are busy, and that reading letters from well-meaning parents about the cause of autism is probably a waste of your time, but I hope you will hear me out. I have heard theories about frontal lobe lesions and brain abnormalities, but I think they are all wrong. My theory may sound far-fetched, but I can't help but feel that I should explain it to someone with your expertise.

In reading about autism I have come across several characteristics of autistic children that are strikingly similar to those of people "tripping" on LSD or mushrooms:

- Extreme self-absorbency
- Insecurity and need for familiarity
- Staring at an object at length
- Self-stimulatory behavior
- Postural insecurity
- Sensory overstimulation

- Inappropriate laughter and irrational fears
- Paranoia and difficulty with eye contact
- Bizarre preoccupations
- Difficulty communicating
- Unusual responses to food
- Abnormal serotonin levels

Watching my son move about the living room, I see an eerie connection. I remember a sort of overwhelming pseudodizziness, a sense of overstimulation that made me feel like I had to shut down for a few moments, so I would lie, facedown on the carpet, until I felt better. I see Miles doing the same thing and I really think I understand why.

Dr. Bauer, please take a moment to theorize on how a child would develop if he were constantly on a neurotransmitter that imitated hallucinogenic drugs. I think learning in normal ways would be extremely difficult for him, and that his world would seem a very different place than ours. I think he would become autistic, and I think the severity of his autism would depend on the amount of neurotransmitter he was producing.

If this is true, wouldn't it be simple enough to cure autism by blocking those receptor sites with an opiate blocker, or with some enantiomeric opposite version of LSD?

Please, let me know what you think of this idea. I hope I haven't wasted your time, or that you can tell me whom else to speak to about this. I would appreciate your keeping this letter confidential, and my husband and I would be pleased to hear from you by telephone, or to meet.

Thank you for your time.*

---

*Stephen Bauer, "Autism and the Pervasive Developmental Disorders," *Pediatrics in Review* 16, no. 4 (1995): 130–36.

THE SIEGE

We're at the mall. Miles and Laura are in a side-by-side double stroller.
They are both getting cranky, but Alan still needs to buy some dress
shirts for work. In the diaper bag are some safety lollipops with looped
handles. They are yellow. I had put them there a long time ago, when
Laura was a baby. Miles looks at his, puzzled. Then he looks at Laura.
She puts hers in her mouth. He does the same. She licks hers. He licks
his. "Alan," I whisper, clutching his arm, "he's watching her! He's
watching Laura!"

Just after his first diagnosis, I had tried several times to get Miles to
do a wooden animal peg puzzle with me. The concept of a puzzle's
purpose was way beyond him. All he would do was remove the giraffe
and run around the room with it. Two weeks later, several days *after* we
took away the milk, he seemed so alert that I tried again. I sat down
with him on my lap and showed him how I could take the pieces out
and put them back in. He showed some interest. I held the giraffe
close to its spot but did not put it in. He reached out and pushed my
hand so that the piece slid into the puzzle.

"Yes, Milo, *yay*! That's very good!" I put the elephant into his hand
and guided it into the right spot. I felt his understanding. We did this
each night, and each night he got just a little bit better. He became
fixated on the giraffe, always wanting to remove and replace it several
times, but I held it firmly in place.

"No giraffe, sweetie. Here's the lion. *Growwl!* Let's put the lion in
the puzzle." I did my best to keep him going. At any hint of abnormal
perseverance I quickly moved things along.

After Miles completed the puzzle, I would let him stim for a few
moments on the giraffe as a reward. Stimming is the abbreviation used
for "self-stimulatory behavior." It is any behavior that the child uses
repetitively to soothe himself. A typical child might fall asleep by twirl-

ing his hair around his finger, or a typical adult might shake his foot while working at a desk. In autistic people such behaviors are abnormal because they use them to extremes. Every hinged object becomes a "stimming toy"; a wheel becomes something to spin for hours. Some autistic kids derive enormous satisfaction from rocking or from twirling their bodies or hands, or, like Miles, from walking on their toes or engaging in repetitive play.

Dr. Bernard Rimland of the Autism Research Institute indicated that he believed the behavior was biologically based. Most experts agree that the behavior must be a physically pleasurable mechanism to relieve stress, and that it may have to do with the release of serotonin into the bloodstream. Higher-functioning autistic adults describe stimming as something that they crave. Those who learn to control such behavior in public find great relief in private moments when they can stim to their heart's content.

Each day Miles was stimming less and less frequently. But he still had no receptive language, and he clearly suffered from "postural insecurity." This was indicated by his caution on stairs, his fear of heights and moving toys such as seesaws, and his frequent loss of balance. When Miles walked or ran, he sometimes looked as though someone just pulled the rug out from under his feet. Before I knew that this had a name, I used to say jokingly that my children were "gravitationally challenged." Now I realized that it was all likely to be part of the same problem.

Actually, Laura exhibited some of the same caution and clumsiness. That made me a little nervous, but it was also comforting. Clearly, nothing was wrong with Laura. Aside from a frequent problem with bad dreams and night waking, her development was all that a parent could hope for. She was kind, patient, and eager to be of help to her little brother. She rejoiced when he did something well, and accepted without resentment the fact that he was getting more and more attention. At three, she could carry on an engaging conversation on a variety of subjects, and seemed to understand that Miles was going to need a special school and special teachers.

I thought hard about everything I had heard about treatment. Since some autistic children are sensitive to sound, auditory integration therapy was developed to ease the confusing signals of the auditory centers. It was thought that this helped such children think more clearly by learning to filter external noise more efficiently.

Sensory integration therapy helped treat postural insecurity in much the same way—by reintroducing tactile stimulation until the child had an easier time handling it. When we met with the service coordinator from Early Intervention (a federally mandated, county-run program that provides services for children up to age three), I decided I would request it with some other occupational therapy. However, it really did not seem likely to me that it could fix the whole problem—only alleviate one of the symptoms.

Behavior modification sounded like animal training. What I had heard made me think it was some inhumane method of controlling the behavior of the profoundly disturbed and severely retarded. There was some reference to the use of "aversives," and I was strongly against looking into this treatment alternative for my son.

That is, until I read The Book.

Catherine Maurice's *Let Me Hear Your Voice* is a poignant, beautifully written book about two siblings who "recovered" from autism because of their mother's dogged efforts and an intensive, home-based behavioral program developed by O. Ivar Lovaas. This was the program that Alan had read about at the library. The two children had apparently recovered fully, and were now "indistinguishable from their peers." Many children had also benefited from this program not by recovering, but by "achieving normal functioning."

As I read, I recognized my son in Catherine Maurice's daughter. Once I was familiar with autism, it was easy for me to see that Miles's behavior was classically autistic. But there is little public awareness about a disorder that, in some form, may strike more than 1 in 400 children. At nineteen months, Miles was one of the lucky few to get an early diagnosis. Most autistic children were not diagnosed until the age of three, even though it is generally agreed that most of those could have been diagnosed at their eighteen-month checkup, using a simple screening such as the CHAT (Checlist for Autism in Toddlers; see Part Two, Chapter 10).

As described by Catherine Maurice, the Lovaas method Alan had read about, the "behavior modification" that I had thought sounded so distasteful, appeared to me to be humane, surprisingly simple, and remarkably elegant. The concept behind the Lovaas method is to break down behavior into small increments, and teach them in small, discrete trials. Each skill must be mastered before moving on to the next one. All of the behaviors that an autistic person does not learn from his environment, such as imitation, language, and problem solving, are addressed in a logical manner. Therapy takes place at a small table, where the child sits facing his teacher.

A child might start with a simple wooden peg puzzle, such as the one I was using with Miles. He would be given one piece, and given the SD (discriminative stimulus) "Do puzzle." He is then prompted— in this case his hand is guided to put the piece in the puzzle. He is then rewarded with a hug, praise, a tickle, a turn with a toy or the lick of a lollipop, or with some other suitable prize. Even though he did not respond alone, the behavior is reinforced.

Next, the piece is given to him again, with the same SD. If he does not respond, the therapist firmly says, "Nope. Do puzzle." The third time the SD is repeated, it is followed by another prompt, then another reinforcer. Soon the child makes the connection between the desired response and the reinforcement, and can do the puzzle piece on his own, after an SD. A good therapist will "fade the prompts" at this point, and eventually fade the reinforcers, so that secondary rewards such as praise and hugs are as effective as lollipop licks, windup toys, and chocolate chips.

Next, a different puzzle piece is introduced. When this is mastered, another. Soon the child may be given two pieces at once, then two different ones, then three, then all of the pieces. The child can now complete the puzzle on his own.

But that is not all he has learned. To a child for whom language is just the movement of other people's lips, this has introduced a simple, clear, understandable command. When the therapist says "Do puzzle," the child understands, perhaps for the first time, what someone wants from him. A window is opened into our world, through which he can see his family and the others around him. If the child and his family are lucky, he might be motivated to look for a doorway.

I could do this. I could see how it might help Miles. Like Catherine Maurice, we had sought out and received an early diagnosis, and Miles was still only twenty months old. This had to be an important factor in her children's success. She had had more money at her disposal than we did, but we were smart and determined. I gave the book to Alan and asked him to read it as soon as possible.

I passed the next few weeks in a haze. Intellectually, I had begun to accept the reality of this diagnosis. But my tears came and went in short, unexpected bursts. I was pushed by a sort of momentum that I knew would keep me from feeling any real pain. As long as there was something I could do, I had power.

I contacted other local parents who had read *Let Me Hear Your Voice* and were doing applied behavior analysis (ABA) with their children. A mom named Shari Rogers spent three hours with me on the telephone and described the efforts of a parents group to make such a program available in our area. Speaking with her about our children was almost euphoric for me. I realized how powerful a bit of support from another parent could be. We were both facing the same indescribable horror, and there was an instant feeling of connection between us.

Shari advised me that since Lovaas himself was a somewhat controversial figure we should call the therapy ABA or "discrete trial teaching." Because these parents had been fighting this battle for the few months preceding Miles's diagnosis, they had made a lot of progress in obtaining appropriate services.

With their help, we lined up a therapist, Jill Pavone, who had some recent experience with the program. Early Intervention agreed to ten hours of home-based therapy, eight hours of special nursery school, and some speech and occupational therapy each week. Much to my relief, I discovered that Miles was entitled to this therapy based on his disability, without any out-of-pocket expenses from us.

All of this accomplished, I lay in my bed one night, using the darkness to map out my plan of action. The program was going to mean an overhaul in our family life. Every spare moment was going to have to be used constructively. I owned my own retail business—two secondhand children's clothing stores—and an increase in payroll would probably eliminate my meager profit, but I had no choice. I would have to give my managers a good raise and ask them to take over most of the buying and administration, and start trying to sell the business. Then I would look into hiring an au pair, a live-in baby-sitter, so that there would always be an adult there for Laura. An English girl who likes doing play dough, I decided. As I drifted off to sleep, I felt confident that I was doing everything I should.

I was in the woods, searching for my son. There was a crackling of underbrush up ahead. I moved quickly, pushing aside branches as the path disappeared into a thicket, then I heard a monstrous roar. Fear gripped me. I couldn't see, but my feet were flying over the ground. Then, suddenly, I tripped and fell hard. I looked up and in the distance saw the outline of a solitary baby boy, toddling slowly toward the sound.

"Oh," I moaned. "Ohhhhh! Oh no!"
Alan sat up in bed.

"What? What's the matter?"

I began to wail. Over and over I howled uncontrollably. As if all of the air in the room was being forced through my body, I howled and howled and howled.

"Karyn, what is it? What's the matter?" Alan asked, frightened. He grabbed my shoulders.

"Oh God, my baby. I'm losing my baby."

"Please, don't . . ."

"My beautiful baby. I cannot bear to lose him." The pain was searing. I cried for Miles, I cried for Alan and myself, and I cried for every family that had ever lived through this nightmare, this anguish, this cruel and perverse torture of watching one's own child disappear into himself.

THERAPY

Six weeks after his initial diagnosis, at the age of twenty months, Miles began his treatment program. His day looked like this:

- Watch *Sesame Street* with Mom and Laura
- Breakfast, school bus
- Specialized nursery school, including speech or occupational therapy
- School bus, lunch, nap
- ABA therapy with Jill
- Snack, play with Laura
- Dinner
- Floor time with Daddy
- More discrete trials with Mommy
- Bedtime

When we watched *Sesame Street,* Laura and I made it as interactive as possible. We participated in songs and counting, constantly spoke about what was going on, and asked Miles a lot of simple questions. "Who is it? It's Elmo! Look! Oscar the Grouch! Oscar is mad at Elmo. What is it? A *horse*! The girl is *riding* the horse. Now she's *feeding* the horse." At first Miles ignored us, but gradually I began to sense that the TV stopped being a lot of moving shapes and became a series of recognizable objects. I watched him closely for signs that a familiar segment or animal excited him. Each passing day I was rewarded by a new glimmer of understanding.

Jill Pavone, Miles's behavioral therapist, was an experienced special education teacher. She was diligent, dedicated, and really seemed to enjoy her work. For the first few sessions Miles screamed a lot, but she patiently held him in his chair and only let him go when the screaming ceased. I was surprised at my calmness, watching him cry. Catherine Maurice had described this, and I remembered reading biographies of Helen Keller; I knew that this gentle discipline was a necessary step for him to be able to learn. I could see how some parents would have a hard time, but I was determined to make this work. Miles was a smart child—he quickly made the connection between being quiet and being released.

"Good quiet," Jill would say. "Good quiet! Go play!"

She let me videotape her sessions with Miles so that Alan and I could watch them each night. Pretty soon I got the hang of the discrete trial format and was able to do some of the therapy myself. We kept track of his progress in a notebook. Jill began with a simple, three-piece shape sorter, with masking tape over the square and triangle. "Do shape," she commanded. Her hand guided his to push the circle through the hole. When Miles mastered the circle, she moved on to the other shapes, one piece at a time. Then she gave him a few pieces at a time, with the SD "Do shapes." In two weeks he had mastered his first program.

It became a joy to see Miles's face when Jill arrived. He would grab her hand and pull her up the stairs, shut the door to his room, and sit at the little table expectantly.

Deep down, I suppose, I still believed that Miles did not have autism. He really seemed to be getting better at a rate that seemed unprecedented. When I asked Jill about this, she hesitated.

"His eye contact is getting pretty good, but I see a lot of other classic delays associated with autism. He's sort of in a class by himself, though. He's picking up speed like I've never seen before."

That was encouraging. If a child *did* recover from autism, wouldn't he be hard to describe? At this point, Miles had most of the delays, but few of the behaviors.

"Jill," I asked, "what would happen if you did this program with a child who didn't have autism?"

"Well, I think it would prove to be rather pointless."

"What do you mean?"

"Karyn, a typical child this age would not need to be taught what to do with a shape sorter."

Alan's time with Miles may have been the most valuable part of the day. As if instructed by an invisible textbook in play therapy, Alan instinctively seemed to know what to do to bring out Miles's awareness of others. He was constantly "in his face," grabbing him as he walked by and forcing him to play "flying baby" or ring-around-the-rosy. He repeatedly initiated "Where's Milo?," which was our version of peekaboo.

At first Miles hated it. He resented this constant barrage of attention and whined to be released. But gradually he began to recognize the pattern of the game, and even smiled when Alan popped out from behind a chair, singing "Where's Daddy? Here I am!"

Another thing that Alan did with him worked in a fascinating way. Using the logic "if autistic children do not point, then teaching Miles to point will cause him to not be autistic," Alan set off on a crusade to teach Miles this skill.

Alan took a flashlight and sat on the floor with Laura. He pointed the beam on the ceiling and said, "Point!" Then he and Laura pointed up. Miles, fascinated by flashlights, seemed to be paying attention.

The beam was turned to the floor. "Point!" They did this several times, and Alan took Miles's hand and formed it into a point when Miles permitted him to. Alan did this every day. On the fourth day, as we all watched, Miles looked at the beam of light on the ceiling and pointed to it. The three of us leapt up with such a roar of praise that Miles was startled. But a smile crept onto his face.

It was strange. Miles now knew how to point his finger but did not understand why he was doing it. The next step was to teach Miles to point at things he wanted. When he was thirsty we always said "Point to the cup" before handing it to him. We would form his hand into a point before he got his reward. It was pure behaviorism, but we were generalizing it throughout his day. He liked cows, and whenever he sat down to eat, we would point to all of the cows in the kitchen, one by one. "Point to the cow! Cow says, 'Mooo!'" The sound of his family mooing seemed to amuse him. Once or twice he pointed, too, and was volubly praised, kissed, and hugged.

"Imitating our pointing isn't really pointing, though," I remarked. Alan had started telling people that Miles could point, but we spent weeks saying "Point to the cup!" without an appropriate response.

Then one day Miles was riding in a shopping cart and spotted a toy cow, and pointed to it excitedly. Alan was so happy, he bought the cow for Miles without thinking twice.

Everything we did seemed to make a difference. Every brief smile that we received was payment enough to keep us going. Every day Miles seemed better.

"It's the therapy," I said. "Just like Catherine Maurice's children, Miles is getting better."

SPECULATION

To the rest of the world, these children pass unnoticed. At best, they are "that strange kid in my daughter's class," or "my friend's niece who re-

cites TV commercials." But there are so many of them, and the number
is inexplicably getting larger.

I would lie awake in bed, mulling this over. What is it about our modern lifestyle that is different? Antibiotics are used a lot more nowadays. Laura was on amoxicillin at least six times in her first year. Miles certainly had had his share. Hadn't I read something about yeast infections being common in autism? Didn't antibiotic use lead to yeast infections? Could this be relevant?

Well, what about chemicals? Cleaning products, air pollutants, plastic cooking bowls . . . could environmental toxins like these be a factor? Autism was first identified in the 1940s, but at that time was considered very rare. Microwaves?

Diet? Well, that has certainly changed. Corn was only brought to European man in the late fifteenth century, and now it's in virtually every prepared food. I knew this because lately Miles was having a mild allergic reaction to a lot of different foods, including corn. I could hardly find anything at the supermarket that he could eat. And only recently had mankind been so enthusiastic about the supposed health benefits of cow's milk.

People were different, too. I had noticed that many highly intelligent people had some mild autistic traits. When two of them got together and had children, perhaps they were more likely to have a child with autism. In tribal times, when spouse selection was much more limited, marriages were likely to be arranged without regard to mutual intellect, but with air travel it is easier for two bright and unusual people to meet at college and later produce offspring.

Then there were vaccinations. I had heard of parents who claimed that vaccinations damaged the immune system and caused their children's autism. I had been pretty skeptical, though. Miles had had reflux, and probably food allergies as a baby. His health had never been vigorous.

I did remember that when he was two months old he had screamed for hours after his DPT vaccination. Alan had rushed home from work to watch Laura so I could take Miles back to the doctor's office—he even got a speeding ticket, frightened by my panicky voice on the phone. The doctor had given me a disgusted look, the nurse had given Miles some Tylenol, and they had both reminded me that this was a common reaction.

Then, at four months old, he was given diphtheria, tetanus, pertussis, haemophilus influenzae B (Hib), oral polio, and hepatitis B, all at once. This time, I gave him plenty of Tylenol beforehand, and after the shots he slept deeply for several hours.

Really, I would describe his development as very normal until about eleven months old. Then, just before Thanksgiving, Miles had a virus that really got him down. Well, we assumed it was a virus, although it did coincide with our introduction of cow's milk. Bright red cheeks, a rash all over his head, face, and neck, a high fever, and another ear infection. Two courses of antibiotics. After that he was cranky much of the time, but definitely not autistic. He still had normal social skills, he just lacked a robust immune system. At thirteen months he could clap hands, play patty-cake and peekaboo, say "cat" and "ish" (fish), and blow kisses. A smart, cute baby.

At fifteen months, Miles had had his MMR vaccine and was sick for several days afterward. That was the week of that Passover dinner when he wound up in the emergency room. In hindsight, I supposed it was then that I thought his development began to slip, and that was definitely when his diarrhea began. But that could be a coincidence. Lots of kids with autism seemed to develop normally for the first year. Twelve to eighteen months was usually the age of onset, when children began to regress, even losing language they might have acquired.

Perhaps the vaccines did coincide with the beginning of the autistic symptoms, but why did Miles have a similar reaction three months later, on the night of his second DPT vaccination?

High-pitched screaming meant extreme pain. Extreme, prolonged pain. I had heard somewhere that this reaction might actually be caused by a swelling of the brain—something like encephalitis. My God, the poor baby, I thought. What if . . . but no. Abruptly, I stopped following that line of reasoning. No, it was practically blasphemy. Vaccines were the best thing to happen to medicine in this century. If they weren't safe, they wouldn't be so widely used.

The books I had read said that autism was neurological, probably due to a structural abnormality of the brain. This had been determined by autopsies of adult autistics that showed abnormalities in the cerebellum. That bothered me, though. If a brain was developing in an unnatural way, for example, if it was subjected to abnormally high levels of some kind of hallucinogenic neurotransmitter, wouldn't it look different after sixty years?

Then again, a brain abnormality kind of made sense. Miles was responding so well to early treatment. His social skills were so much better, it was hard to believe he was the same child. Could he be stimulating his neurons to adapt to his disability? Were we actually teaching him *how* to learn?

One afternoon, soon after the day he had mastered the simple shape sorter, Miles began to shut down. Jill brought him downstairs early, explaining that she thought he might be sick or need another nap. After she left, he began to whine and cry, and then spent fifteen minutes stimming on the Sit 'n Spin toy. I was alarmed and I did not know what to think. Had all of this progress been temporary? He woke up screaming from his nap again, for the first time in weeks. By midafternoon, our newest baby-sitter, Jean, tapped on my office door. She was so agitated by his fussing that she asked to leave for the day.

I decided not to say anything to Alan when he got home, since he took everything related to Miles so hard. I hoped he would not notice. But he did.

I was making dinner and Alan was watching the kids. After five minutes he stormed into the kitchen. "What is the matter with Miles?" he demanded.

"I don't know," I replied. "Maybe he's getting an ear infection."

"He doesn't get those anymore."

"Well, maybe he's getting one now."

"He's not turning to his name, and I can't get him to look at me. He's been walking on his toes since I got home, and now he's stimming on the Sit 'n Spin. He hasn't acted like this in weeks." Alan's eyes looked very dark.

"I don't know, Alan." I tried to keep my voice level. I knew it was easier to keep him calm if I underreacted in a crisis. "We can't expect him to have a good day every day."

But this was worse than a bad day. Miles had reverted to his autistic behaviors, stimming on everything he touched and dragging his forehead across the wood floors.

Neither of us slept well that night. The next morning, as I dressed him for school, Miles seemed better. Alan phoned three times from work and asked me to describe his behavior.

Later, when Miles got off the bus, there was a note in his schoolbag from the teacher. As I read it, I let out a cry.

I forgot to let you know—Miles got hold of a piece of cheese yesterday morning. When we realized, he had already eaten most of it. Sorry!

CHAPTER THREE

The Importance of the Diet

REVELATIONS

I bought a modem and I am on the Internet. I do not really know how it works or what it's for, but if it's the Information Superhighway then there might be something here about autism and the use of dairy products. Newsgroups—Autism. How does this work? Oh, I see. Someone posts to the group and the others reply. Well, let's give it a try. "Could my child's autism be caused by MILK?" They're going to think I'm crazy.

When we had removed dairy products, Miles's silence had changed to language that consisted of a constant stream of meaningless jargon. It sometimes sounded like real language, or like a foreign language. His voice rose and fell melodically, but the words were unintelligible.

After Miles had mastered some basic imitation, such as clapping his hands, patting his head, and touching the table, Jill decided that it was time to begin verbal imitation. She asked me to list some of the "jargon" words that I had heard him use. Miles had some verbal stims that he repeated over and over, such as "ah-shoo." She began with that one.

"Miles, say 'ah-shoo.'"

Hearing the word sometimes made him repeat it.

"Ah-shoo, ah-shoo, ah-shoo . . ."

"Good boy! Very good!" Jill gave him a reward of a small windup toy. She let him play with it for a moment, then began again.

"Say 'ah-shoo.'"

"Ah-shoo."

"Hooray! Nice work! Take a break, buddy, go play!"

Listening on the baby monitor, I smiled. I could see where this would lead, and I knew that Miles would someday be able to use language. It might take years, but he would do it.

In only a few weeks, Miles had several real words under his belt. The first ones to appear were "cat" and "fish," the words he had lost. Then came "cow," "moo," and "hat."

The next program gave meaning to the sounds. The jungle animal puzzle resurfaced as a language tool. Jill would hold up the giraffe and say "What is it?" When Miles approximated the word, he was given the puzzle piece and allowed to place it in the frame as a reward. His word acquisition picked up speed: "tiger," "lion," "monkey." His pronunciation was terrible—"aya-shoo" for "elephant"—but we did not care. He was learning to talk.

Since Miles was so fascinated by animals, Jill concentrated on those words at first. When she tried to slip in words like "Mommy" and "Daddy," Miles just looked at her blankly. I longed for the day that Miles would call me Mommy. I even fantasized about it. Now that he was off milk, anything seemed possible. The difference in him was astonishing.

Since the day that he ate the cheese at school, a lot of puzzle pieces had begun to fit into place. We had switched from soy formula to cow's milk at eleven months old, just before the mysterious "virus." Miles's ear infections had begun at that time, too. Come to think of it, lots of kids were switched to cow's milk at about a year, the age when autistic behaviors commonly began to emerge.

I called Shari Rogers, the mom who had been so helpful in helping us set up our ABA program, and was surprised to learn that several other parents in my area had their autistic children off dairy products. They reported an improvement in eye contact that made it worthwhile. No one seemed to be having the results that we were, though. I guessed that this was because we had stumbled upon the answer so early. The average age of diagnosis was more than three years. By that time parents were only just finding out about the idea of dietary intervention, months or years later than we had started with Miles.

We were lucky. Miles was diagnosed at nineteen months, and taken off dairy two weeks later. If this was the reason he was doing so well, then time was clearly a critical factor. The urgency of learning more about this became apparent to me. How many children like Miles were at an age that their abnormal brain development could still be reversed? How could they be identified?

Shari had taken wheat out of her son's diet, as well as dairy. She told me that there were a lot of reports of autistic children responding to a dairy-free, wheat-free diet.

"Well, milk seems to have been most of Miles's problem. Thank goodness I don't have to worry about a wheat-free diet, too. Mostly all that Miles will eat now is pasta and pretzels."

"Oh, I know. Jack craves bread, too. It's really hard for him to see his brothers eating it when he can't have it."

There was that word "crave" again. Miles had craved milk before we took it away. Why did he crave pasta so much nowadays? The previous night he had eaten three large bowlfuls at a sitting. Since he had been off milk, he had stepped up his desire for anything containing wheat. Could this be a problem for him, too?

I was so busy I refused to consider this possibility. Miles was progressing very well, and supervising his intensive behavioral program was a lot of work. My main concern lately had been over his chronic diarrhea. Miles ate nothing but rice, chicken, pasta, bread, and french fries cooked in canola oil, yet his bowel movements had gone from being loose to runny to diarrhea, every day. We called him "the amazing exploding baby" and had to change his clothing frequently. It had a pungent, sour smell, contained large particles of undigested food, and looked decidedly unhealthy.

Our pediatrician dismissed this with "some children just have loose stools." I asked her if she would look at his messy diaper once, but she refused. She told me that this was called "chronic, nonspecific diarrhea." So, if it had a name, I guessed it was supposed to be okay. But it was not okay with me. Every symptom must have a cause. I asked for a referral to a gastroenterologist.

I remembered that I had posted my question about milk on the autism list the day before. How long was I supposed to wait before checking my e-mail? Perhaps someone had replied.

I sat down at the computer and got on the Internet. I was eager to see if anyone on the Autism Newsgroup had answered my query about milk. I noted with excitement that I had some e-mail, but when I pulled it up, I was not prepared for the response. To the question "Could my child's autism be caused by MILK?" there were forty-one messages in my box.

THE INTERNET

Would I do anything for my child? What would I risk to save a stranger's child? Will I fight this thing, beat it down until it exists no more to torture innocent families? This goal will become part of my life, my daily purpose, my reason for living. I have no choice. I will be driven in a way that I never dreamed I could, and I will not rest until the beast has been slain.

I was not the only parent to take this secret oath. I'm sure other parents of children with other disabilities besides autism have taken it, too.

But as far as my mind could imagine, there *was* no diagnosis worse than autism. Down's syndrome seemed like a blessing in comparison. People with autism often suffered from terrible fear and frustration, frightful outbursts of temper, migraines, seizures, and worst of all: self-injurious behavior (SIB). There is nothing worse than watching a child smash himself in the face until bruises and bleeding appear. In my opinion, an affectionate, loving family member who made gains slowly was far better than a child whose greatest gains would barely, if ever, lead him to any kind of self-sufficiency, or any kind of satisfying relationship with his own parents.

And the dreaded cancers and leukemias, how much worse could they be? The memory of a child who had a short but happy life seemed better than a lifetime of caring for a child suffering constantly from anxiety and discomfort, who panicked at any change in routine, who needed a great deal of care and gave little in return. At the time Miles was diagnosed, it seemed to me a nightmare, a death curse, a daily torture of immense proportions, both for the child and for his family. I had been told that Rain Man (the movie character portrayed by Dustin Hoffman) was a "best-case scenario": an example of "high-functioning" autism, and I hadn't yet met the families whose children were surpassing these expectations.

Perhaps the bleak outlook was why parents of children with autism had already done a phenomenal amount of work and research toward understanding and curing this disability. In fact, almost every big name in autism research I'd heard of had an autistic person in their family.

The response to my posting about milk finally convinced me that Miles had something more than an allergy or misdiagnosis. Parents of autistic children from all over the world had seen results ranging from mild to dramatic after implementing this diet. Many of them used the expression CF/GF, meaning casein-free/gluten-free. Casein is a milk protein and gluten is a wheat protein, found in wheat, oats, rye, and barley. Apparently, the two proteins are structurally very similar.

Parent 1

My son had several undiagnosed food allergies, among them were wheat and dairy products (basically everything he normally ate was harmful to him). He has been on a wheat- and dairy-free diet since October, and I can see a noticeable difference in his verbal skills.

Parent 2

When traces of gluten get into his now rigorously gluten-free diet, he acts drunk. And with casein he becomes psychotic-looking, not autistic, but absolutely hallucinating out of his mind. His younger NT [neurotypical] brother immediately becomes constipated with the slightest trace of milk or cheese. What do all of those processes have in common?

Parent 3

My son's doctor suggested we modify his diet to remove anything that would promote yeast growth (sugars) and potential allergens (wheat, dairy, corn, citrus). She took blood work at that time to check all sorts of stuff. When we returned three weeks later, he was much improved, his tongue didn't have that whitish look, the dark circles under his eyes had cleared, and the yeasty bumps on his backside had disappeared. He was much calmer and more focused.

Using his blood work, his doctor prescribed supplements to help correct his nutritional deficiencies: iron with vitamin C for anemia, B complex, and a multitab of vitamins A, E, C, and zinc. She also suggested that we add in one at a time all of the potential allergens. He had problems with everything but corn.

It is amazing, when he gets any sort of a milk product, he gets an ear infection within three days. We treat them a bit differently now. If we catch it early, we treat it first with a prescription decongestant/antihistamine with no added sugar or dyes and echinacea. We only use broad-spectrum if it is more advanced (you really need a pediatrician you can trust here). When we do use antibiotics, he takes nystatin (an antifungal medication) four times a day while he is on the antibiotics.

He still is on a restrictive diet, which means I need to send his food with him almost everywhere he goes, but that is a small price to pay. His behavior and communication skills have improved so greatly that after the initial three weeks I have had no problem getting the school and the day care to cooperate. As far as trying to quantify the changes, his language has improved greatly. He now is beginning to understand contractions, "wh" questions, and pronouns! Behaviorwise, he can actually sit in one place for more than thirty seconds—even people who know us casually have commented on how much his behavior has improved (people at church—yes, he can actually sit through a whole service!), people we play baseball with, doctors who see us one or two times a year. . . .

Anyway, sorry for being so long-winded, but I hope this gives you a little picture of what I've seen. If you want more information, recipes, my doctor's name if your doctor wants to consult with her, more information on what we've done for supplementation and why, just drop me a note.

Parent 4

I no longer believe in cures, but I do believe in improvements. I also believe that there are different causes for autistic behaviors. My son is very gluten intolerant and his behaviors deteriorate drastically when he gets it. I think each individual has to try what they feel they can if there is no harm in the program. We have had success with AIT [auditory integration training], prism lenses, main-streaming, diet, and other therapies. Not a cure, mind you, but Dan, age twenty-one, is getting a regular high school diploma and has his first competitive job doing data entry for a local store. He is working ten hours a week and will go to full time this summer. Don't give up or condemn everything if it hasn't worked for you. Not everything we tried worked either, but if you have a success, it is well worth it.

That sounded like good advice. It seemed that those who had actually tried the diet were enthusiastic about it. Its critics all seemed to be those who refused to try it. A father named Roy posted the following:

At last, a panacea for autism! Join the ranks of Lovaas and "Bears & Suzi Kaufman." Those of us who have been dealing with the cure-alls and miracle makers for fifteen years or more can only be amused at first, then saddened by so simple an attempt at THE CURE for, perhaps, the most pervasive disorder in the world. If it were as simple as eliminating certain foods from our children's diets, do you think organizations, newsgroups, research, etc., would still be necessary? Or, was this a slightly delayed April Fool's joke?

I felt sorry for this person. We were seeing firsthand the success of a Lovaas-type approach and the dietary intervention. If he did not think these things could work for his child, perhaps his child was different from mine. It was obvious that his level of despair was different from mine, too. I strongly believed that with every passing week that he was left untreated, Miles's symptoms would have been harder to reverse. Perhaps Roy's window of opportunity was too tightly shut. Hope gleamed from every crevice of ours. I said yet another silent prayer of thanks that Miles was getting better.

But what if the cause of *most* cases of autism was strongly linked to diet? It is not impossible to believe that certain foods could cause certain reactions. If individuals with phenylketonuria eat foods containing phenylalanine, they will suffer brain damage, and sometimes even end up with *autism*. Celiac disease, I had recently learned, was a disorder that caused people to become sick from eating the food protein gluten.

I was interested in celiac disease (CD) because it often resulted in chronic diarrhea, which Miles still had, and because it had to do with gluten, this food that some parents of autistic children were eliminating from their diets. It was a disorder in which the intestinal villi, the little hairlike projections that line the intestine, are flattened from a reaction to gluten. This makes them unable to absorb essential nutrients from food. Treatment requires a lifelong, strict, gluten-free diet.

In addition, celiac disease interested me because I had heard that it could affect you psychologically as well as physically, causing poor mental functioning, or brain fog. Such reactions generally occurred shortly after eating gluten, which made me suspect that it was affecting the brain in some immediate way.

Celiac disease was usually diagnosed after a patient had experienced serious, long-term diarrhea, or after other GI (gastrointestinal) problems. Most medical doctors are taught to look for classic symptoms like chronic diarrhea or constipation, or both; or abdominal cramping and foul, frothy, or floating stools. However, some patients with CD had vague, varied symptoms like headaches, bone or joint pain, depression, weakness, or fatigue, while some were virtually symptom-free. Sometimes it went undiagnosed for years until a sharp-minded physician decided to run a battery of tests.

Since the disorder is usually screened with a blood test for "endomysial and gliadin antibodies," which is not terribly accurate (especially if the subject is already on a gluten-free diet), a "small bowel biopsy" (where a piece of the lining of the small intestine is taken by endoscopy, a minor surgical procedure) is often necessary for the diagnosis. Many doctors are not familiar with the disease, and frequently take no further steps after a negative blood test. Therefore, although it is estimated that at least 1 in 250 persons in the United States is affected, celiac disease is grossly underdiagnosed.

Unfortunately, the results of leaving celiac disease untreated over a long period of time can be serious, causing iron deficiency anemia, bone or dental disease and osteoporosis, severe vitamin deficiencies, pancreatic insufficiency, or intestinal lymphomas.

Although I had never heard of celiac disease before, I certainly should not have been surprised by the connection between food and physical well-being. My mother suffered from crippling arthritis at the age of forty that turned out to be an allergy to nightshade foods: tomatoes, potatoes, eggplant, and peppers. Her instantaneous recovery baffled her doctor, who was more inclined to call the problem psychological than he was to admit the possibility of food allergy. Over the years I had seen the odd slipup, when she ate some ketchup or a few french fries, and I knew how bitterly she regretted it the following day.

Even I had a lactose intolerance, and it was not until I was seventeen that a doctor showed enough concern about my chronic diarrhea to suggest that lactose—milk sugar—might be the culprit. But most doctors think of food as the last possible cause of a medical problem—it is not part of their training. My sister Sylvia, a physician in Oregon, told me that courses in nutrition are not a requirement in most medical schools.

It surprised me that Miles's doctors were not more curious to find a cause for his problems, rather than just treat the symptoms. Miles had been diagnosed and treated for a whole list of "disorders" without the slightest thought about their origin. This list was quite long when I wrote it out. He had been given the following diagnoses, which were really just descriptions of his symptoms:

- Reflux
- Sleep disturbances
- Asthma
- Ear infections
- "Glue ear"
- Eczema
- High fevers
- Seizures
- Chronic nonspecific diarrhea
- Language delay
- Autism

Well, I had seen the effect of milk on Miles's autism with my own eyes. If his doctors did not care about the cause, then I would look for it myself. The Internet was a powerful tool.

I could only wonder whether Roy's son could have responded the same way to dietary changes if his father had not given up hoping. One of the other parents answered him with this comment:

> Roy, many people have seen marked improvement in their children's behavior when they have changed the diet. There is a great deal of evidence that many autistic children are also gluten intolerant. No one is claiming this will "cure" autism. But many kids have been helped by this noninvasive, SAFE intervention. It amazes me that a parent would take this attitude without doing a little bit of background reading. If you want to chalk this up to quackery without trying it, fine. But don't discourage others.

I made a note of this articulate parent's name: Lisa S. Lewis. It seemed to me I had heard that name before, but I could not remember where.

I spent hours on the list, reading the archives, and wondering about the connection between autism and dairy. There was a lot of anecdotal information but nothing concrete. "Anecdotal" means that an effect has been observed but not scientifically proven. Two of my siblings and several of my friends were doctors—I knew how doctors think. Without double-blind studies, nothing a parent claimed had any credibility. I myself had no evidence to prove that the connection was real, aside from my observations about Miles's improvement, and his deterioration when he ate dairy. But at least I was not alone. On the Internet, a mother named Chris Braffet Delnat wrote:

> My son has been gluten- and casein-free for about a year now, and it has been the best year ever. He is no longer aggressive, ever, and no longer has wide and wild mood swings. His nocturnal bowel movements and the consequent feces smearing is gone; his compulsive eating and consequent weight problem is also no more. He is now able to go shopping with me and go about in the community without bolting away or screaming. He is growing tall and slim and looks healthy.
>
> What has not changed are his tactile defensiveness, what appears to me to be a visual field integration problem, and verbalizations remain limited.
>
> His activity level has gone down, down, down, until now he has to be encouraged to do something other than sit on his bed looking out of the window. Quite a change from the whirlwind of activity that kept me exhausted just one year ago and a new cause of concern. Clearly, his difficulties are tied in with his particular metabolism of foods.
>
> My fear is that I've not identified all that is doing damage to his system and that his life could somehow be improved if I would only figure it out. It would help immensely if the mechanisms by which the gluten and casein proteins cause problems were definitively identified; perhaps we could extrapolate from that point.

That's what I wanted to know. What were the mechanisms that were malfunctioning in these children? Later, Chris described her experience in greater detail:

Occasionally I post my son Andrew's progress on the gluten- and casein-free diet, which he has been on for over one year. I thought this might be a good time to do it again, in light of some list members pooh-poohing the idea that diet could possibly be of any value.

When I started my son on the diet we were at the bottom of a downhill behavioral slide with nowhere else to turn. Andrew had been excluded from school for aggressive, uncontrollable behavior and I was with him the majority of the day, one-on-one, just to keep him from hurting himself too badly.

He was at a point where he could maintain some semblance of composure only in the security of his own room. He was fourteen years old, 185 pounds at 5' 8"; a big boy who sometimes would bowl over whoever was standing in his way.

He had wide, wild mood swings, would become panicked easily, and was generally very difficult to handle. I had stopped taking him out except when absolutely necessary for fear that he would get the urge to leave the car while it was rolling down the street, not to mention having to frequently sprint after him in parking lots, stores, etc. The school was recommending a hospitalization in a children's psychiatric ward. He was on Mellaril and had been on Prozac prior to the Mellaril. He was miserable, and I was in agony over not being able to find a way for him to lead a life with even a marginal quality of existence. We were pretty low, all alone, with no help in sight.

I read about the diet here, on the list. Jean Jasinski . . . bless her kind and caring heart . . . sent me copies of Reichelt's 1991 article out of *Brain Dysfunction,* as well as urinary peptide testing info. Lisa Lewis sent me her personal archive of the previous discussions in 1993 of the diet and some notes of encouragement. I read this stuff, decided that it was worth a try, and went all out. The first thing that happened was my poor boy, already distressed, went into a ferocious withdrawal. We were one-on-one in his room for about a week. He tore himself up, tore me up, and it was horrid. I'd read that this happened some of the time with Reichelt's subjects, so I was not surprised (only very haggard) and was actually heartened by the knowledge that I had probably hit on *something*. There had to be some reason for a withdrawal that fierce, so Reichelt's opioid excess theory became even more rational to me. After about a week Andrew started to calm—down, down, down, he came. He slowly but surely became calm, cool, collected, and such good company. Within the space of two months he was more level, more attentive, more social than I had seen him ever before.

During all of this I utilized the due process procedures to put together an educational program that would benefit my boy. Yesterday we had his summer IEP [individualized education plan] meeting. Everything is going along so well. This has been by far the best year ever for Andrew and his progress astounds even me. He has learned to swim laps in the pool; has started a new job recently (wrapping silverware at a local nursing home); can go anywhere in the community safely with an adult; patiently pushes the shopping cart for me in the store, stopping when I ask; seeks out the company of both me and his sisters at home. In short, he's doing marvelous.

He definitely is not *cured*. He still has autism. He has tactile defensiveness (much less severe now), remains functionally nonverbal (dramatic increase in appropriate nonverbal communication skills though), still gets anxious when routines are disturbed (although he is much less dependent on routine now), and has a processing delay.

In the past year his quality of life has increased dramatically with the removal of the stress that the gluten and casein was putting on him. He appears happy, even playful at times, he is no longer aggressive toward others, he no longer tears his fingernails off or even picks at his fingers, he no longer has nocturnal feces smearing, he is no longer incontinent of urine during the day (a periodic problem before), and he no longer eats compulsively. He also has no need for any medications of any sort. The only thing he takes are gluten- and casein-free calcium and magnesium supplements, a B_6 supplement, and a multivitamin. He is growing. He has lost forty-five pounds. He is a tall, lean, 140-pound handsome young man.

The quality of life for the whole family has taken a dramatic turn for the better. I was able to leave him with a respite provider for eleven whole days last month to go to Hawaii to get married. I was able to return to work last fall to pursue my career as an advocate for community support for people with disabilities. My daughters can bring friends over and they're not terrified of what their brother may do. Most important, Andrew feels better than ever before. I have finally found a way to help him. He's got so much potential now! It's a far cry from the looming specter of the in-patient unit full of lost souls doing the Haldol shuffle!

This is Andrew's story. I realize that only a portion of children with autism will probably benefit from this diet, for it would have to be part of their particular problem. Autism is so diverse in its etiology. My deepest regret is that I didn't find out ten years earlier and halt the inexorable damage done as opiates wreaked havoc in my beautiful son's brain. So I urge all of you to at least investigate this as a possibility for your own children.

I was amazed. But what did she mean by "Reichelt's opioid excess theory"? Who was Reichelt, and what kind of research had he done about autism and diet? I had to find out as soon as possible.

Finally, about a week later, I read something posted to the autism listserv (the online discussion group that I had joined) by Paul Shattock, a researcher at the University of Sunderland in England.

It is impossible to cover all aspects of research in a single posting so, like all arrogant researchers, I will concentrate on those aspects that I find interesting. Those in our own group are unashamed subscribers to the "opioid excess" theory of autism as first enunciated by [Jaak] Panksepp. He was struck by the similarities between the "symptoms" of autism and the effects of opioids on animals.

I remembered my letter to Dr. Bauer, which had never been answered, and became excited. So I was not the only person who suspected that there were mind-altering drugs at work here!

I knew a little bit about opiates from a brain chemistry course I took in college. Opium, derived from the poppy plant, was used for years as a painkiller, and endorphins are opiates that occur naturally in our bodies and are released during stress as painkillers, as well as at times of heightened excitement. Opiates are highly addictive in any form.

Reichelt suggested that the source of these "opioids" could be peptides that result from incomplete breakdown of certain foods, in particular casein from milk and gluten from wheat and other cereal products. It has been demonstrated that if casein or gluten are mixed with stomach enzymes, opioid peptides (known as casomorphins and gluteomorphins) will result. Normally, these would be broken down further into individual amino acids, but if the appropriate enzymes are not present or are otherwise inhibited, the peptides will persist and could get out of the gastrointestinal tract and into the blood.

This was exciting! It meant that if something was wrong with Miles's digestive system, or if certain enzymes were missing, milk and wheat proteins could be turned into opiates.

> From here, the majority will be dumped in the urine, which is where Reichelt, ourselves, and others find them. Some could enter the "brain," where they could either have direct opioid activity themselves, or so swamp the body's natural enzyme systems that break down our natural opioids (endorphins), that these persist and exert their effects. These effects will include disrupting neurotransmission in all of the main systems (dopamine, serotonin, GABA, etc.). Consequently, perceptions by all of the senses (hearing, sight, taste, proprioception, pain, etc.) will be affected to a varying degree. At the same time, so will the ability to filter out what is important from what is not. These opioids constitute an important element in the immune system.

I had to read this passage three times to understand what it meant. Essentially, it said that these opiates, if they are permitted to enter the brain, can have a widespread effect on the nervous system similar to that of hallucinogenic drugs; and this results, in a developing child's brain, in autistic behaviors. The proof of this lies in the presence of such drugs in the urine of the autistic children.

> The brain and the immune system communicate by means of chemicals, of which opioid peptides form an important group. Depending upon their concentration, they will either stimulate or inhibit the immune system (a gross oversimplification for which I apologize). Anything that either increases or reduces the availability of these peptides to the brain could influence the symptoms seen. Amongst these one should mention the activity of sulfur transferase enzymes ("pests," as they tend to be called on this list).

The consequences of lower than normal PST [phenol sulfur transferase] activity are many, but would include such things as abnormal breakdown of serotonin (and certain drugs as well), and reduced breakdown of bilirubin and biliverdin that could be evidenced by the dark rings we see around the eyes of some people with autism. Most important, in our opinion, would be the increased permeability of the gut. Theoretically, even if the peptides are present, they should experience some difficulty in getting out of the gut and into the blood. The lack of S-transferase activity would result in increased permeability of the gut.

If there is an already low activity with PST, anything in the diet which requires PST activity could exacerbate the situation. Oranges, apples, tomatoes, etc., are prime examples, but any food with these phenolic compounds could have the same effects. The problem is that it is not possible to avoid phenolic compounds in diet. They occur in virtually everything.

So, there might be other foods involved, as well. This caught my attention because oranges, apples, tomatoes, and red grapes were among the foods to which Miles was severely reactive. All gave him hives or a severe diaper rash, ever since his diarrhea had started. Was this a coincidence, or did he indeed have a problem breaking down phenolic foods?

A couple of other observations relevant to comments which have recently appeared on this list:

1. The abnormalities reported in the cerebellum and corpus callosum (Courchesne) and the Purkinje cells (Bauman) are consistent with continued exposure to opioids.

This was what I had suspected: that the brain abnormalities found in adult autistics' autopsies could have been acquired, not inborn.

2. The increasing incidence in the developing world may be reflective of an improvement in diagnostic procedures, but it could also reflect the introduction of Western diets, which are heavily dependent upon wheat and milk.

3. The incidence of candida in the intestines and elsewhere may or may not be significant in the causation of autism. Personally, I keep an open mind on that one. However, it should be noted that such organisms, which would normally be controlled by the immune system, could flourish where the immune system is compromised. The presence of the candida could be a consequence of repeated antibiotic use, but it could also be a mere epiphenomenon.

Candida was a species of yeast. Although I had repeatedly heard that there was some relationship between yeast and autism, my brain was so full of information that I was not yet ready to follow that train of thought.

4. The common but not universal history of ear infections and insertion of grommets ("ear tubes" in the U.S.) could similarly be indicative of a compromised immune system. It is commonly an "allergic"-type reaction to milk (again epiphenomenal).

Well, this might be merely anecdotal, but it was certainly true of my son!

5. Certain infections would influence the permeability of the blood brain barrier so that materials that may be in the blood and would normally be kept out of the sensitive brain tissues would, subsequent to certain infections, permeate much more readily than before. Many parents report the first signs of autism immediately subsequent to an infection (encephalitis, for

example). For this reason I respect the observations of parents who comment upon the effects of vaccines on their previously "normal" children.

"Encephalitis" means "swelling of the brain." I knew it had been theorized that this is what causes the high-pitched screaming seen after vaccinations. I didn't want to think about it, but once again I had to remind myself that Miles's autism had begun after his MMR vaccine.

If this is true, what can be done?

1. Avoid gluten and casein.
2. Some parents have experimented with digestive enzymes (personally I would plump for bromelain on theoretical grounds) but I have never heard any results either positive or negative with such therapies.
3. Attempt to encourage PST activity (using epsom salt baths).
4. Avoid all foods with phenolics, or at least those with appreciable quantities.
5. It has been suggested that people with disorders related to autism (specifically dyslexia) suffer from a deficit in the ability to convert linoleic acid to gamma linoleic acid. This is required for (amongst other things) an intact gut wall. Providing GLA would, under these circumstances, be beneficial.

I appreciate that many will already be familiar with much of this story, but it may be news to others. I would recommend Lisa Lewis's WWW page for anyone interested.

Paul Shattock

This was so exciting I could barely stay in my chair. I forwarded the information to Alan's computer at work and left him a message to read it as soon as possible and to pick up some epsom salts on his way home from work.

Lisa Lewis was the parent who had stuck up for dietary intervention on the autism list. I made a note to look for her web page.

When I was in college, the best professor I had was Terry Hines. He was a member of the Psychology Department and taught classes in experimental psychology, brain physiology, and "Pseudoscience and the Paranormal." He later published an excellent book by that name. I took every class he offered. It was his emphasis on careful experimentation that had kept me objective when watching for changes in Miles. He also taught us how to evaluate everything we heard or read before deciding if it was true.

One thing that Professor Hines had warned us about was a "nonfalsifiable hypothesis." For example, if I were to say that I had just created the world and everything in it last night, you might challenge me with "But I remember going to a picnic last week." I could reply that I created your memories of the picnic. In fact, I could easily account for any argument you might have. With a nonfalsifiable hypothesis, one cannot imagine a way to disprove it. If I claim to have ESP but fail to show it in a series of tests, I can say that the laboratory setting makes the effect go away, or that the presence of a skeptic makes it go away, and there is no test you could do to prove me wrong.

Nonfalsifiable hypotheses were to be treated with great suspicion, and were usually the mark of "pseudoscience." Dr. Hines couldn't think of a single example of one that was proven to be true. I challenged him on this: "What about the theory of evolution? If I say that the graceful neck of the giraffe is nothing less than an act of God, you can simply explain that evolution made his neck longer to reach the acacia leaves at the top of the tree."

"Ah, but we can *imagine* evidence which would disprove the theory. If a new species of deer is found with a solid gold femur, on which the Ten Commandments are inscribed, I would be the first to say that the evolution theory is incorrect. On the other hand, there is no evidence imaginable that would convince the 'psychic' that his theory has been disproved."

Paul Shattock's explanation of this "opioid excess theory" seemed to account for every physiological abnormality that was common to children with autism, and some of them simply couldn't be proven yet because there were no tests available to do so. But I *could* imagine clinical trials whose results could *disprove* the theory, such as testing the levels of casomorphin in the urine before and after the diet was implemented. If it could be disproved, this also meant that it could be proved. Either Shattock was right, or he was wrong. Science would one day find out.

I wrote a long summary of Miles's history and e-mailed it to Shattock. The next day I eagerly read his reply. He called Miles's story "a bit of a classic" and congratulated us on coming upon this information so early.

We corresponded a lot after that. Paul was not a physician, but over the years he had heard feedback from a lot of parents of autistic children. He was a charming, knowledgeable person who always took the time to answer our questions in detail.

He had suggested that we try removing gluten from Miles's diet, indicating that it might control his diarrhea. He pointed out that the casein and gluten proteins were so similar that if one had been a problem, the other should also be removed. He referred me to an Internet newsgroup for people with celiac disease for information about implementing the diet. I joked that if Miles had a normal bowel movement I would buy Paul a bottle of champagne.

GLUTEN

I called Shari Rogers, the mom who had helped me with the ABA program, to let her know that taking Jack off *wheat* was not enough, according to what I'd read. Gluten could be found in wheat, oats, barley, *and* rye, and was added to most packaged foods as a filler. She took the news calmly.

"Just when I thought this diet couldn't get any harder," she said with a sigh. I knew exactly what she meant. The diet meant more research, more study of a new topic, and my brain already felt like it was crammed with information.

At our appointment with a pediatric gastroenterologist, I brought Miles's diaper from that morning, and was relieved when she agreed to look at it.

"Whew, that looks like diarrhea to me. His diapers always look like this?"

"That's not normal, is it?"

"No, that's not normal. Has Miles lost any weight?"

"Just in the last couple of months—he's lost about three pounds."

"I don't know what to make of it. I've never heard of autism linked with a gluten intolerance, but I'd be happy to look at the research if you forward it to me. I'm going to order tests for celiac disease. You can take him off gluten if you like, but if the tests are negative, I'll be really surprised if it makes a difference. Please let me know what happens."

As an afterthought, I asked her to prescribe nystatin for Miles. There was all that stuff about gastrointestinal yeast on the Internet. Nystatin is a harmless enough medication, so although Dr. Brown looked doubtful, she gave me the prescription.

Two days went by, then three. There was no change in the amazing exploding baby. At breakfast one morning I decided to give up on the gluten-free diet. It was just too difficult to maintain, Miles was barely eating, and I hated having to read labels so carefully. Thinking this, I absently read the side of the Rice Krispies box.

"Malt flavoring. I wonder what that is. Could that have gluten in it?" I got on the celiac listserv and posed my question. Five minutes later I had an answer.

Barley malt did indeed contain gluten, if not very much. I pulled out a bag of puffed rice—I would give the diet one more day.

Jean, our baby-sitter, was really excited about the change in Miles. He was not quite two years old. He almost never cried now, and was becoming more delightful every day, chattering away with his sing-song jargoning and bringing us toys to look at and share with him. When she got to my house the next day, I ran out to my store and then did some errands before returning home.

"Jean? I'm home. I brought some fries for Miles; did he eat lunch yet? Jean?"

Jean walked up to the door with her eyes dancing. She was holding a diaper behind her back and she presented it to me like a rare jewel. "Look," she said. It was a perfectly formed stool, Miles's first in months.

We paged Alan at work to tell him the news. I doubt that in the history of mankind three adults had ever been so excited about a dirty diaper. I added a bottle of champagne for Paul to the increasing tally of our financial deficit.

Despite this good news, I was extremely stressed, and I knew that I was in over my head. Never a terribly neat or organized person, I had recently been losing my grip on the task of running my household, leaving bills unpaid and paying dozens of overdraft fees and late fees, and missing appointments more often than keeping them. I never stopped moving—flitting from one task to the other, distracted by the pile of mail, the ringing phone, the mountain of laundry, the tapioca cookies I had promised to bake, the demands of running two retail stores.

I had customers with two-year-old twins, *and* one-year-old triplets. Five boys under three. Everyone marveled at their fortitude, but I secretly wondered if my life was harder than theirs. Regardless, I had discovered that self-pity was a useless waste of time. On the phone, our family members were sympathetic, but they didn't realize what we were going through, and many were dealing with problems of their own. We had no relatives in town. There was no one to give us money or support. There was no one who could help us, so we had to do the best we could.

I wished that Alan could have done more, but he had become crippled by anxiety, stepping over the trash bag on his way out of the door, losing his desire or ability to tidy up after himself or the children. He had lost his father the same month that Miles was diagnosed and was doing the barest minimum to maintain himself. He seemed so fragile that I tried to do more and more to make things easier for him.

Only Laura seemed fine, but I knew that the long-term effect of the situation would take its toll on her, too. At three and a half she was perceptive enough to know that something about her parents had changed.

Luckily, our search for an au pair had been rewarded. From the moment I picked up her written application, I knew that Cheryl Ostryn was exactly what we needed. I had looked at my watch, calculated the time difference from England, and phoned immediately. My instincts were correct. Cheryl was a very bright girl who was looking for an adventure: a year in the United States. She and I were on the same wavelength: we "clicked." She reminded me of myself at eighteen, and I knew that having her in our house would be an advantage, not an intrusion. She proved to be a hard worker who knew how to handle responsibility.

I explained as much as I could about Miles, without using the word "autism." Had he still actually appeared autistic, I would have had to tell her the truth up front, but he was clearly not functioning like an autistic child, and I was afraid of frightening her off. Although his language was severely delayed, he was very easy to supervise and care for. Later, after Cheryl had met the children, I told her the entire story, and she was amazed.

Aside from being a charismatic beauty with a cascade of flaming red curls, Cheryl was a natural with children. Laura adored her from the beginning, and Miles accepted her quickly as another primary caretaker. Cheryl was swiftly able to understand how to generalize Miles's therapy into his daily routine, and improved upon our efforts with energetic creativity.

Cheryl was able to keep the children on a schedule, give them their vitamins and medications, keep them entertained without the television, and give them appropriate attention while I was away. She reminded me about doctors' appointments, Miles's groceries, and the various tasks that were required from parents by the chirpy little notes that came home in the children's backpacks. In short, she brought stability to our household.

Of course, Cheryl's salary was almost exactly what I was now earning from my business. But having another adult in the house was a blessing and a relief.

"Do you think that removing gluten from Miles's diet has made a difference in his behavior?" she asked.

"I don't think so. Do you?"

"It's hard to say. He seems to be progressing so fast that it's hard to judge whether it has made a difference."

"That's what I think. Well, at least he doesn't have diarrhea. That alone makes it worthwhile. One of the moms on the Internet told me that her son responded more slowly and less dramatically to the removal of gluten than he did to the removal of dairy, and that it took longer to see an effect."

"Well, I don't mind doing it. Just be sure to label those biscuits— those cookies you're making, so I know they're okay for Miles."

When I finally figured out how to look for websites on the Internet, I found Lisa Lewis's paper, entitled "An Experimental Treatment for Autism." I discovered that Lisa had had the opposite experience with her son, Sam, who was doing very well on the diet, but appeared to react much more radically to gluten than casein. Apparently, it had to do with the child's subtype of the disorder, the amount of dairy or gluten he was eating before the diet, and other mysterious factors.

I wished I had found her paper sooner. Aside from including food lists with warnings about things like barley malt, and other dietary questions that I had finally answered through extensive research, it contained in twenty pages the same information that had taken me months to discover. I made a note to get in touch with Lisa, whose quest for knowledge had been much like my own.

Alan and I really did not know if the nystatin was having an effect either. We had been seeing some good language development. For example, once when Miles pulled on my hand, I asked, "What do you want?" He pointed with one finger and replied, quite clearly, "This balloon!"

Miles seemed to be improving at the same rapid but steady rate we had seen since the removal of dairy products from his diet. Then something unexpected happened.

I was packing Miles's schoolbag and I found a note from his occupational therapist, who saw him at school and had no idea about nystatin or the change in his diet.

> Miles's balance and coordination have improved dramatically in
> the last two weeks. He allowed me to pull him on the wheel board
> and does not seem to be falling down nearly as much.

"Cheryl, come here a minute. Does Miles seem less clumsy than he used to?" We went into the living room and watched Miles trot across the room.

"Now that you mention it, yes he does. Quite remarkably so."

I realized that he looked sure-footed, even graceful. The sudden staggers and swervings were gone. When had this happened? His postural insecurity had disappeared. Just like that. The next day, for the first time, he went up the stairs on his feet instead of on all fours.

Now my belief that I had some control over Miles's condition was confirmed. I became obsessed with finding more answers, and with convincing everyone that I had found the secret to curing at least one subtype of autism. But I was to learn that it was not going to be that easy.

The difference in my son from the day we took him off dairy had been spectacular, astonishing, and unmistakable. If we had not tried taken this path when we did, I shuddered to think what he would look like then, or in a year, or in a decade. I urged Paul Shattock to pursue his research. If the results were conclusive and a routine test could be developed, just imagine the generations of children who could be helped, and the parents who would no longer be forced to come to terms with this diagnosis of a "severe, lifelong disability" for their beautiful, intelligent children.

At that time, it seemed to be simple enough to describe Miles's autism as an enzyme deficiency or a metabolic disorder. That may yet turn out to be the simple truth. But the one thing that I was to learn was this: whenever I thought I understood the problem, I was about to discover just how much I did not know. Every month, as my research continued, I would look back with derision at my ignorance of the previous month. This was very humbling. I learned that however much one knew about autism back in 1995, one still only knew part of the story.

I also learned that an open-minded parent with an autistic child and Internet access could learn more about the biology of autism than a closed-minded clinician with twenty years of experience in developmental disabilities, and that other parents were a better resource for practical advice than professionals.

Lisa Lewis turned out to be one of the few parents who knew more about the disorder than I did. When I complained on the autism listserv that I wanted a different name for the disorder, since my son no longer acted autistic and I didn't know how to describe his illness, she reminded me that for most people the disease and the symptoms were the same thing.

I took her criticism hard. Perhaps she was right. Still, although I saw her point, I wondered what would happen in the future when the disorder did become fully understood. What if it was possible to diagnose and stop the disease process *before* it resulted in the autistic behaviors? Could you still call a person with the disorder "autistic"? I thought not. Paul Shattock replied to this question by agreeing with me, but pointed out that, like phenylketonuria, the ultimate name for the disease would eventually come from a better understanding of its cause.

However, Miles *had* lost his autistic behaviors, yet he still had the disease that caused them.

Dear Lisa,

My son was taken off of the offending foods after a very limited exposure and is almost fully recovered (totally declassifiable as per top experts) four months after his diagnosis (which was a real low point). This is why, in my (subjective) opinion, the food sensitivities caused his autism. I know beyond all doubt that in another six months the damage to his development would have been irreversible.

Perhaps Miles has a subtype of this disorder that has a more defined causality—I don't know. My instinct is that other autistic kids with allergies have something very much the same, or similar.

It is simply illogical to me that children with autism should so commonly have a recurring pattern of food intolerance that we consider to be a mere symptom. Especially considering the all too common story of normal development until twelve months of age, when foods like cow's milk and wheat products are frequently introduced.

My puzzle is what to call my son's disorder. His social skills are now normal, and autism is no longer descriptive. However, on a typical diet, he would certainly exhibit autistic behavior and development. I really have to say that Miles has a disorder involving a global intolerance to various foods, affecting his brain as well as his body.

Perhaps someday we'll know whether or not that is the actual definition of autism.

So, for the time being, there was no name for the beast. It would have been so nice to say something to a new doctor like "Miles has Reichelt's disorder" and have her understand what it meant. Luckily, Dr. Hyman, Miles's developmental pediatrician, seemed to be taking us seriously, and encouraged us to document Miles's progress and record any behavioral changes as we experimented with his diet.

Unfortunately, Miles's pediatrician, Dr. Stover, had moved away, and I was back to square one in the search for a regular pediatrician. This time, I was in a real bind.

Being in a managed care medical program (an HMO), I discovered an unsettling truth. Most private practice pediatricians don't accept new patients. They will accept newborns, but routinely turn away children who have left other practices. Presumably, this is because an older child in search of a new doctor is highly likely to have a health problem that will require greater effort and possibly a referral to a specialist—something that HMO doctors are discouraged from giving. My only option was to go back to the medical center and take my chances in the "pediatrician potluck."

CHAPTER FOUR

Science's Questions, My Answers

THE YEAST CONNECTION

Why were some kids responders to dietary intervention, showing dramatic results right away, and others slower to improve, or hardly improved at all? Somehow, I suspected that when I knew the answer to that one, the puzzle would finally be solved.

I assumed it had to do with age and length of exposure, but I knew a little girl named Larisa, just Miles's age, who had been off dairy since she was fifteen months old and showed only mildly improved eye contact. She was later taken off gluten, and her response to that was also apparent, but not significant. She still seemed, for all the world, like a child on a high dose of LSD.

I had somehow become the local dietary guru for other autism parents, but I was still at a loss for so many answers. I pondered the mysterious issues I had read about on the Internet: yeast, vitamin B, phenols, salicylates, glutathione, EPD, essential fatty acids. Miles was doing very well, but I worried that I'd kick myself later if by neglecting these items I was hindering his recovery. I saw these as other symptoms of the dietary intolerance, not as a cause of autism per se. Miles clearly had bowel and behavioral reactions to most foods high in phenols or salicylates, including peanuts, soy, corn, eggs, tomatoes, dark grapes, and apples, but in the interest of maintaining a balanced diet I used some of them in moderation. Were these opioid-linked, autism-inducing, or just an example of his body's nasty tendency to malprocess food?

My local chapter of the Autism Society of America had decided to sponsor a conference. Bernard Rimland was the keynote speaker. Also scheduled were an occupational therapist, and a pathologist named William Shaw. The ASA president knew that I was researching diet and other biological interventions, so she kindly offered to let me chauffeur Dr. Rimland to the conference and then later drive Bill Shaw to the airport.

I remembered reading something about William Shaw. Something about fungal metabolites in urine. I looked forward to hearing his talk, since anything regarding the etiology, the *cause,* of autism was more interesting to me than theories about treating its symptoms.

Dr. Rimland was the head of the Autism Research Institute in San Diego. He was the hero of every parent of an autistic child I knew. He was the psychologist who, back in 1964, wrote *Infantile Autism,* the book that concluded that autism was not a psychological disorder caused by unloving mothers but was neurological and physiological. His son Mark was an autistic savant, an excellent artist, and had inspired his father's dedication to this field.

It was ludicrous that autism was once thought to be psychological and that autistic children were once subjected to psychotherapy, with the implication that parents had somehow traumatized their children into this condition. I could not imagine being burdened with such guilt in addition to the shock of learning that I would be raising a child with autism. Dr. Rimland had done a great service for the families of these kids and for me, and I subscribed to his newsletter, the *Autism Research Review International.*

Today, as I do, Dr. Rimland believes that autism is a treatable biological disorder, but the medical community does not. No amount of parent testimonials has changed what they think they know. I thought about the fable about the blind men and the elephant—how one grabbed its tail and said that elephants were long and skinny, like a snake. Another grabbed its ear and had quite a different impression of elephants.

So it was with autism. A psychoanalyst might look at an autistic person and say, "Aha! Childhood trauma." Tests show abnormal neurological development, and the neurologists might say, "Aha! Neurological." Autistic people whose brains had been subjected to abnormal neurological development for decades were found at autopsy to have an abnormal cerebellum. The physicians might say, "Aha! Congenital! A structural abnormality." The geneticists, finding a pattern of abnormal sequences in the DNA of autistics, might say, "Aha! I have found the autism gene!" I wondered if perhaps what they were finding would turn out to be an "autoimmunity gene" or an "allergy gene."

But a parent is the one person who sees the whole child and who watches his transition from a reasonably normal baby into an autistic toddler. Those who try the biological intervention know exactly what changes they are seeing. When I asked one of my physician friends why she thought Dr. Rimland had lost credibility with the medical community, she shrugged and replied, "Probably because he's not a doctor, he's a psychologist. Besides, he's a parent."

This was true; Dr. Rimland did have a son with autism. That this was held against him was a sad reflection on the perceived levels of competency of the American parent, and of the arrogance of some doctors. I appreciate the fact that physicians are trained to protect their patients from unproven quack remedies, since laymen may lack the scientific judgment to protect themselves. But I suspect that there are occasions on which the advancement of medicine has suffered as a result.

There is currently an upsurge of interest in alternative therapies: drug-free approaches to illness that include nutrition, supplementation with vitamins and herbal remedies, exercise, pain management through meditation, massage, and other interventions. These treatments are usually harmless, may produce some clear benefits that even doctors cannot dispute, and do not put billions of dollars into the pockets of large pharmaceutical companies, which, incidentally, spare no expense in wooing physicians to use their products.

Still, with Professor Hines's spirit constantly supervising my forays into the hypothetical, I was very careful about my opinions in this area. Always a firm believer in classical medicine, I never had the urge to pass up a known medical treatment for one that was untested and anecdotal. For all of my righteous indignation, I still knew one thing for a fact: *If there were a safe drug that effectively reversed the symptoms of autism, I would certainly have chosen it over diet.* The drug companies could have my business, and I would not have to rearrange my kitchen, my schedule, or my life.

I called the Autism Research Institute and spoke with Dr. Rimland. He was a lovely person to talk to—warm, astute, and extremely concerned about the welfare of an entire community of disabled people who had been thrust into his keeping. He knew what I knew about the effect of diet on some children and was pleased to hear that Miles was doing so well.

However, he was frustrated at the slow pace with which this current research was moving. He told me that he had predicted ten years ago that the information on the malprocessing of casein and gluten would be common knowledge by now. But it was not.

I admitted to myself that I knew why this was so. Traditionally, physicians see the people who run out to the health food store to try a new herbal remedy or homeopathic cure as crackpots. In fact, I had to admit that they often were pretty flaky. Many of the people who had previously pitched ginseng, melatonin, beta-carotene, algae, and high-dosage vitamin C in my direction had ranked very low on my credibility list, and I was aware that people sometimes died of treatable diseases because they had chosen meditation over chemotherapy.

Then again, the medicinal herb echinacea had recently achieved substantiation from reputable researchers as a legitimate immune system booster, and after years of relative obscurity was now gaining widespread popularity. I had tried the herb and was pleased to find that it seemed to be effective in reducing the duration and severity of cold symptoms. The mechanism for its effectiveness may not be clearly understood, but reputable double-blind, placebo studies had shown that it does work.

Dietary intervention for autism was much the same. There had to be a reason why this worked. Granted, the research was only preliminary, but it was a safe intervention and could at least be recognized until more data had been collected. A great deal of what we know about medicine had begun with anecdotal reports. Why was this so different?

I guessed I knew what had occurred. When information first began to be released about a dietary intervention for autism, the first people to run out and try it were the flakes. When it worked, the medical community had to listen to a bunch of flaky people running around shouting "Oh, why is no one *listening* to us?" Instantly, the whole idea lost its credibility, and was relegated to pseudoscience. Little interest or funding was available to create good studies, and the issue has been suffering ever since.

Was I becoming a flake? I hoped not.

For the first time, I began to wonder how many other ideas I had dismissed because they were unproven. Who was to say that some of them were not just as valid as ones that had been proven?

Alan brought home some research papers from a Dr. Dohan dating from 1949, describing studies in which children with developmental delays responded dramatically to the removal of certain foods from their diets. Dohan was so convinced of this issue that he spent his entire career trying to prove that it was true, but never gained any real recognition.

Dr. Rimland was a big proponent of vitamin B_6 and magnesium supplementation for autistic people. At least one biological subgroup did not seem to be utilizing their B_6 very well, and supplementation made a big difference for those individuals. Personally, I did not see a difference in Miles when we tried a product called Super Nu-Thera, which was a high-dosage vitamin powder rich in B_6 and magnesium. However, I knew many parents who said they did, and I believed them. Rimland had a good point—if it's harmless and might help, why not try it? An observant parent should be able to tell if it makes a difference.

I was excited about meeting Dr. Rimland. In Catherine Maurice's *Let Me Hear Your Voice,* the man had nearly been deified. As a parent of an autistic child, I was inexpressibly grateful to him for overturning the view that autism was psychological.

On the morning of the conference I was up early. I cleaned out my car, packed up my briefcase, and left myself plenty of time to get to Rimland's hotel. When I turned my key in the ignition, however, nothing happened. I let out a shriek. Almost in hysterics, I ran into the house and phoned Alan.

"Come home, I need your car!"

"Karyn, it's a total mess."

"But he's waiting for me outside the hotel—I have to go now!"

Alan's car was indeed a mess, rusted on the outside and filled with dust, crumpled paper, and soda cans. By the time I reached the hotel, I wasn't very late but I was a nervous wreck.

As it turned out, Dr. Rimland was kind, sincere, and friendly, like a favorite uncle. I tried to calm down, but I found myself babbling.

Never one to pay much attention to movie stars or other famous people, I realized that I was starstruck by a middle-aged psychologist. He took this in stride, and was even very kind about the fact that I got completely lost on the way to the conference.

Dr. Rimland's lecture was entertaining and informative. He talked about vitamin B_6 and magnesium, and about the fact that physicians consistently ignored studies, no matter how well designed, that showed any benefit from vitamin supplementation. We shared a lot of the same opinions about this. I had found over the past few months that most physicians selectively chose only the studies that supported already held beliefs about food allergy and ignored most others.

I watched a bit of the presentation from the occupational therapist. She was showing a video of a child doing Lovaas therapy while jumping on a trampoline. His speech improved when he was in a heightened state of arousal. His food reinforcers were little cheesy Goldfish crackers.

As much as the discrete trial therapy and the physical therapy had helped Miles to catch up, neither of them would have been one-tenth as effective if he had not been on the diet. I simply knew this to be true. On the rare days when he had been contaminated with dairy, or even corn or soy, Miles's therapy was a complete waste of the county's money.

Perhaps the child on the trampoline would not have responded to the diet. But treating the symptoms of autism without attacking the cause was difficult for me to watch, and I left the room.

Later, when Bill Shaw finally got up to speak, I held my breath. Please, let him not be a crackpot.

He stood at the podium and gave an apologetic grin. "When I first heard about gastrointestinal yeast," he began, "I didn't give it much thought. My opinion of the 'yeast people' was that they were the same folks who claim to have been abducted by aliens."

The crowd laughed. I let out a slow sigh of relief. I took careful notes so that I could be sure of understanding what he was saying.

Candida exists in two forms: yeast and fungus. Normally, in our gut, we have some of the yeast form of candida. These are kept from becoming too numerous by some of the naturally existing healthy flora, probiotics such as lactobacillus and bifidobacteria, also known as acidophilus.

If you think of your lawn, you can understand what's going on. The grass (acidophilus) and the weeds (candida) are competing for space. If a blight (antibiotics) attacks only the grass, the weeds will take over.

Antibiotics selectively kill off our "good-guy bacteria" while ignoring the candida. This is why some people eat yogurt (which contains probiotics) when they have a yeast infection or while they are on antibiotics. When the teams get unbalanced, the "bad guys" take over and become numerous.

A healthy immune system will control candida with its natural antibody system. If it doesn't, and the candida has been around for a while, it can turn into its fungal, or mycelial, form. This is barbed, toxic, and difficult to kill. One theory proposed that this form of candida slowly pokes holes in the intestinal wall, causing gut permeability, or leaky gut syndrome.

I later read an article about leaky-gut syndrome.* It explained that a healthy small intestine allows only nutrients to pass into the bloodstream, typically blocking out larger products like incompletely digested fats, proteins, starches, and bacteria. However, when the integrity of the gut wall has been compromised, the body, recognizing these as foreign substances, triggers an immune response. The proponents of this theory claim that for those likely to suffer from this condition, good health can be restored by healing a leaky gut with strict diets and nutritional supplements like the amino acid glutamine—the fuel intestinal cells use to replace themselves.

One of the theories about how the gut lining becomes compromised is that bacteria and yeast overwhelm it and migrate into the

---

*Wendy Marston, "Gut Reactions: Leaky Gut Syndrome," *Newsweek,* November 17, 1997. "Tiny leaks in the lining of the small intestine may play a role in diseases as diverse as asthma and arthritis."

bloodstream. Other possible causes are a compromised immune system or a parasitic infection. An overview of the subject published in 1995 in the journal *Gastroenterology* found increased evidence of leaky gut in diabetics and schizophrenics, among others. Dr. Douglas Wilmore, a researcher at Harvard Medical School, showed how intestinal permeability increased in postoperative patients and people with AIDS.

Dr. Shaw explained that this may be the means by which large food peptides like casomorphin and alpha-gliadin were leaking into the bloodstream, which would explain why children like Miles responded to a dairy- and gluten-free diet!

I knew from the Internet that this could be occurring in autistic children because there were many who had very abnormal results on gut permeability tests. Such tests were usually done on people with celiac disease, the severe gluten intolerance. I wondered whether the gut permeability could be caused either by the candida or by the gluten, and result in the same problem with milk and wheat. Perhaps one type of autism *is* some form of celiac disease?

Another danger of having too much gastrointestinal yeast is that it seems to interfere with mental and physical function, especially when it dies off. This feeling of discomfort can cause the subject to crave sugar, thus keeping the little parasites alive and healthy.

In a normal individual, yeast overgrowth should not occur. As I mentioned earlier, part of our immune system is set up to control the yeast in our bodies. However, in people with a compromised immune system, such as those with cancer or AIDS, candida can become a real threat to the individual's health.

If a young child is born with an immune defect, or with a slight susceptibility compounded by long-term antibiotic use, it is conceivable that candida could get a stronghold in his gut. If candida was present early in his life, a child's immune system's "memory" might mistakenly assume that its presence is acceptable and refrain from making antibodies. I had started Miles on nystatin without really understanding much of this, but now I realized why it might be effective. If his chronic antibiotic use for ear infections had allowed yeast to poke holes in his small intestine, this might have been the beginning of Miles's disease process. Or, if his immune system was compromised, the presence of yeast could simply be making a bad situation worse.

Bill Shaw was a legitimate scientist and, much to my relief, did not appear to be on the lunatic fringe of medical science. His interest in autism had begun a couple of years earlier, when he was working at his lab at Children's Mercy Hospital in Kansas City, Missouri.

Part of his job was to test for inborn errors in metabolism. One day, when using some new mass spectrometry equipment, he noticed unusual peaks in the urine of two brothers. When he inquired about these substances, he was told to ignore them. They were fungal metabolites, or the waste products from yeast in the gut. Since they were not human in origin, they were generally disregarded.

Shaw wondered about this. A few weeks later, when he was again testing the urine of the two brothers, someone mentioned to him that the brothers were autistic. When Shaw checked his database for the results of the tests of other autistic children, he found the same peaks. What was going on here? What was all this yeast doing in the stomachs of children with a neurological disorder?

At that time Bernard Rimland had already received hundreds of reports of autistic children improving while on nystatin or other antifungals. Shaw discussed this finding with him, then decided to do a study and publish his work.

I liked Bill Shaw. He was intelligent and easy to talk to. He was not the parent of an autistic child, and putting himself in a class with the "yeast people" was politically a very dangerous thing to do. I regretted that the trip to the airport was so short.

After the conference, I ran my ideas by Alan, who frowned as he sat down to think about the yeast connection.

"It may be candida, or it may be another organism, something like an anaerobic bacteria. The nystatin may be doing something different than you think. It might be working *in* the bloodstream."

"But how could it?" I asked. "Nystatin is nonsystemic. It works in the gut and is not absorbed into the bloodstream."

"Okay, but think about it. If there is a leaky gut, it *could* be getting into the bloodstream."

"I didn't think of that," I said, marveling at Alan's insight.

"Shaw may be right. All I'm saying is don't jump to conclusions. You'd be surprised to learn how many medications used to treat gastrointestinal problems have neurological effects. Still, I do think we should keep Miles on the nystatin." He sighed. "I just wish someone had done a really good clinical trial."

At about the same time that Miles was diagnosed, Rimland was pulling together the DAN! (Defeat Autism Now!) Conference. The result of the collaborative efforts of the researchers who attended was a manual called the *DAN! Protocol*. It was an instruction book on what biological tests were useful in treating children with autism, and hypotheses on what was going on.

It seemed that there was a familiar biological pattern that many of these children were following. In a simplified outline, the process goes something like this:

1. Children may be born with a genetic predisposition toward food and other allergies.
2. And/or, at some point in their development, a "viral load" such as a triple vaccination or a case of roseola or the chicken pox may trigger an abnormal immune response.
3. The child becomes ill and is given antibiotics.
4. The candida in their intestines then transmutes into a nastier

version that attacks their gut, causing changes in the GI immune system and a leaky gut.

5. This is seen with the malprocessing of certain proteins, such as casein and gluten. Instead of being properly utilized, they are broken down into neurotransmitters, which affect their brains.

This explanation was still a bit sketchy, but it fit in with what Paul Shattock had written. I decided that Step 2 might occur after Step 4. If true, it helped to solve some mysteries, such as the observation that some children with autism improved on antiyeast medications. Miles had started taking nystatin at the same time he was taken off gluten, so we were not sure if his recent acceleration was due to any or both of these factors. Perhaps the yeast was causing some sort of drunkenness that accounted for his lack of balance, or perhaps it was the gluten, causing him to "trip" on opiate imitators. What we really needed was a doctor who knew something about this disorder and could tell us what to do. But there was no such doctor in my city. In fact, we still hadn't even found a new pediatrician. For the time being, it seemed, our most powerful weapon was my computer.

On the Internet, we heard about some doctors who had set up specialty practices dealing with this unnamed phenomenon, many of whom were "environmental physicians." They firmly believed that autism was an environmental illness. Since its prevalence was increasing, this was likely to be true, but environmental physicians had strayed from the medical fold and I wondered if they were likely to be taken seriously by doctors such as Susan Hyman.

Some parents swore that a doctor in Los Angeles had helped their children, while others had misgivings—one complained that he was doing some interesting but expensive and unnecessary testing on his autistic patients, and routinely prescribing drugs for them such as Prozac and Ritalin without fully exploring the avenues of dietary or biological intervention. How could I judge doctors like this? There simply was no established medical protocol for dealing with the biological cause of this disorder.

There were a few other physicians investigating this area of medicine, but many seemed to be ordering expensive tests that had no treatment implications. During the conferences I attended, I became friendly with Bob Sinaiko, a physician in San Francisco, and Jeff Kopelson, another, in Brewster, New York. Neither had autistic children, but both were willing to risk their careers by recommending safe, alternative treatments for their patients with autism.

We did not know if there were other doctors closer to our home, or if there were, how we would pay for their services. Miles's illness was quickly taking us to the brink of bankruptcy, and in our managed health care plan, out-of-state physicians were rarely covered. I had started my business because we had had staggering student loans to pay off, and now my absence at the store meant loss of income, which meant that we were steadily relying on credit cards for groceries, gas, and other necessities.

Until we could find a professional who would help us solve Miles's problems, we had to rely on our instincts. Like so many other parents who had had success treating the biological cause of their children's autism in addition to the symptoms, we were on our own. Our objectivity was put to the test many times. It was important to both of us to be sure of what we thought we knew.

"Karyn, I think this new potato drink mix, this Vegelicious stuff, is making him kind of edgy," Alan once said. "He's been cranky for the two days he's been on it."

"But I really like it—it has the same amount of calcium, with a lot less sugar than the rice milk. Maybe something else is bothering him and it's a coincidence."

"I think it's the beverage."

"Maybe he's coming down with a cold."

"Beverage."

"Maybe it's not the new stuff, but withdrawal from the rice milk. He has been kind of addicted to that lately."

"Maybe."

There was a suspicious ingredient in Vegelicious near the very bottom of the list—corn solids. I called the company, and Fred, the marketing manager, insisted that this was an insignificant amount of corn.

I tested the drink on three separate occasions, one of them when Alan was unaware of the test. Each time Miles did become unusually cranky, so we threw the rest of it away. A month later Fred phoned me to say that they had removed the corn from the ingredients and were now calling the product DariFree. We bought some more, pessimistically tried it again, and were surprised to see no reaction. The drink turned out to be a favorite in our household, a staple that both children loved and which was delicious in baked goods. When we ordered it in bulk, it was even the same price as regular milk. There were small blessings sprinkled throughout the ordeal of doing this diet, and finding a good milk substitute was one of them.

We never again deliberately "challenged" Miles with casein or gluten. However, we were given the opportunity to be certain that gluten had been causing his diarrhea. Two days before we left for Florida to visit my mother, Miles picked up an animal cracker from the floor at school. His teacher was changing another child's diaper and watched helplessly as Miles put the whole thing in his mouth. Miles then cried almost continuously for forty-eight hours and suffered from terrible diarrhea for days. My mother remarked that he seemed unusually cranky during our trip, although it was hard to say whether this was caused by the change in his environment, by stomach pain, or by an actual mental reaction to the gluten. We refused to make assumptions based on speculation. Regardless, we tightened our control over his exposure to breadcrumbs or any traces of gluten. I devised a homemade play dough concocted from rice flour and sent a pound of it with Miles to school. (See Part Two, Chapter 13.)

Two months later I stopped at Burger King on the way home from an appointment with my ophthalmologist and picked up some fries for Miles. They fried their potatoes in canola oil at that time, and Miles tolerated them. I was having great difficulty focusing my eyes because of some drops the doctor had given me for an eye test. When I got home, I gave Miles the packet and watched him eat about half before I noticed that the printing on the package looked different.

What had I recently read on the Internet? Something about Burger King. Oh yes, they were going to be introducing new fries containing gluten (from wheat) and whey (from dairy) in certain test cities.

I grabbed the packet away from Miles and held it up, but I simply could not read what it said.

"Laura, come here."

"What, Mommy?"

"What does this say?" Laura was almost four and she knew her letters.

"N-E-W." She smiled proudly. I tried to stay calm.

"Good, that spells 'new.' What are these letters?"

"R-E-C-I-P-E. What does that mean?" I felt a chill.

"It means that Miles probably can't have these fries anymore."

Sure enough, Miles was once again contaminated with gluten. This time there was no question about his reaction. The diarrhea started just after dinnertime and continued for six days. Jill complained that his therapy sessions were a complete waste of her time. After six days of constant tantrums, apparent headaches, and an unprecedented obsession with dinosaurs, Miles woke up cheerful, with a normal diaper.

We now felt with much greater certainty that we knew what we were seeing, and more than ever I wished for a pediatrician with whom we could discuss our observations. The one I had met at the medical center, Miles's fourth in his young life, was an instant disappointment. Almost immediately, she started giving me what I called "the Weird Look." Unfortunately for me, she had had some experience with autism during her residency and therefore *knew* that what I was saying could not be true.

Just when I was ready to accept the situation, Jill Pavone provided the solution to our problem. One of the things she sometimes did with Miles was to walk with him to the library and let him pick out a book, pointing out people, objects, and actions along the way. I happened to stop in while they were there, and found Jill talking with a tall, attractive woman with intelligent eyes, who was introduced to me as Mary Beth Robinson, a pediatrician.

She commented that Miles was a charming child, and was surprised when I told her briefly of his history. Miles reached for me to pick him up, and smiled at her shyly from my arms.

"I have several autistic patients," she said. "I've actually heard of this diet before."

"Ah. Well, how open-minded are you about it?"

"I trust parents. If they tell me that they believe something, I respect that it is likely to be true."

I smiled.

"Are you accepting new patients?"

A month later, I arrived at Dr. Robinson's pediatric practice alone, for a consultation. At the reception desk I was amazed to be handed a booklet with her group's philosophy, their strong belief in the teamwork of parents and physicians, and each of the doctors' home telephone number. When I was shown into the office, Dr. Robinson welcomed me warmly, and pulled out a notebook.

"Tell me all about Miles," she said. And I did, pouring out every detail of his history for almost an hour, expecting to be cut off with an impatient word. But I was not. Dr. Robinson listened carefully, taking notes, interjecting occasionally with questions or comments. She slowed me down and asked for more details when I went too quickly or skipped parts of the story.

I felt my growing excitement as I spoke. Dr. Robinson believed me!

She had heard the story and was impressed and interested, not irritated and dismissive. She wanted to help Miles. She wanted me to provide her with any materials that she might read about diet and the biology of autism. I was almost in a state of disbelief. Finally, after a thorough discussion about what tests we planned to run, and what kind of treatment Miles might need, we stood up and shook hands.

"I have a question," I said, with a nervous smile.

"Sure, what is it?" she replied.

"Are you a real doctor, or is there a TV camera in this office?"

She laughed. "I really prefer to practice medicine this way. I am a parent myself, with four daughters. That is the kind of humbling experience you don't get in medical school."

These words made me realize how prejudiced I had become about the medical profession. There were good doctors to be found, if one was persistent enough.

Soon several other families with autistic children switched over to Dr. Robinson's practice, and we were encouraged by the fact that each of us provided her with experience that would benefit us all.

I had learned another lesson, an important one: You have the right to use a doctor who shows you respect and listens to your observations. You should feel comfortable teaching her what you know and learning from her expertise and experience. You should have confidence in her judgment not because she has a medical degree, but because you know her to be fair as well as responsible. You should be able to trust her not to ridicule your ideas and to give you all of the information you need to make intelligent decisions. If you cannot, then it is *your* responsibility to find another doctor.

LET ME HEAR YOUR VOICE

Our efforts were really paying off. In six months Miles had gone from an autistic child with no language and poor adaptive skills to a delightful little boy who was pointing to objects he wanted, putting two words together appropriately, and initiating games like peekaboo and ring-around-the-rosy. He ate with a spoon, helped get himself dressed, and named hundreds of objects around the house. His language was becoming easier to decipher now, too. Even strangers could understand most of it.

I had spoken with Dr. Susan Hyman on the phone a few times, and we had worked together on a committee to help implement more appropriate educational programs for children with autism. Dr. Bauer was on the committee, too, and smiled indulgently when I explained that I was the parent who had written the letter about hallucinogenic drugs.

"Are you aware that opiate blockers have been tested on autistic children?" he asked. "Your observations were interesting, but the results of giving naloxone to autistics were not very promising. This leads me to believe that autism is *not* due to an opiate problem."

"Well, maybe not completely, but there has to be a reason why my son improved when taken off those foods." I then filled him in about my research, Paul Shattock's work, and Miles's progress. "You don't believe me, do you?" I asked, recognizing the Weird Look as it crept across his face.

"I believe that *you* believe it. But no, I don't believe that diet has anything to do with autism."

He was a nice man, and I couldn't dislike him for his honesty.

"Okay, then we'll agree to disagree," I said, smiling. "Someday, one of us will turn out to be right, and one of us will turn out to be wrong." He smiled, too.

Susan had seemed pleased to hear of Miles's improvement, but clearly did not understand the extent of the change in him, so the following week I sent her a videotape. The tape was about ten minutes of Miles playing with Laura, getting a tiger ride from Alan, and playing peekaboo and giggling with me.

She phoned me that night after the kids were in bed. "Karyn, I am absolutely floored. I just watched the tape and my mouth was hanging open the whole time. I am really impressed with the change in him. What I saw was not an example of autistic behavior." She agreed to come visit him soon.

Dinosaurs had become an interest of Miles's. Actually, I had to admit that they were an obsession. He knew them all by name, and sometimes did a little bit of verbal stimming on the names: "Tywann-isauwus wex, Tywannisauwus wex, Tywannisauwus wex, Tywannisau-wus wex . . ." We did not take away his dinosaur toys, however, because his play with them was so normal. He would use two toy dinosaurs to enact a conversation, playing both parts. When speaking for the dino-saurs, his language was a mixture of jargon and real words, sometimes in short, meaningful sentences.

"Hi, you a Ceratops?"

"Aha. I Ceratops."

"Roaaar!"

"Roaaarrrr!"

I joked to my friends that he could name every dinosaur but that he still couldn't call me Mommy.

One day at the shopping mall Miles and Laura were running around some benches, hiding then popping up. When Laura jumped up from behind her bench, Miles waved at her.

"Hi, Waw-waw!" he shouted. Alan and I looked at each other excit-edly. Laura simply responded, "Hi, Milesie!"

Another time, on an airplane, Miles was absorbed with a book and did not notice Alan leaving his seat. When Miles looked up, he looked at me and clearly asked, "Where's Daddy?" I stared at him for a moment, wondering if he had really said what I thought he had said.

"Daddy will be right back," I replied hesitantly. Miles went back to his book.

Just a few days later, I was sitting in the living room watching Miles play. He was looking through some cards with dinosaurs on them. When he got to his favorite one, he became quite excited. "Wook, Mommy, wook at dis. Issa Tywannisauwus wex."

I sat, stunned for a moment, and then I began to weep. At twenty-eight months old, more than twice the age his sister had been when she evidenced the same knowledge, Miles knew that his mother had a name. I held out my arms and said, "Miles, come here. Come to Mommy."

He put down the card and stood up with a big smile. He ran into my arms with an expression of pure joy, and when I picked him up, he wrapped his arms tightly around my neck. It felt so good to hold him without being pushed away. As if he knew how I was feeling, he let me hold him like that for a long time. A long, wonderful time.

For months an old poem had been dancing along the fringes of my mind, and suddenly a scrap burst forward:

And hast thou slain the Jabberwock?
Come to my arms, my beamish boy.

Miles then lifted his head from my shoulder and gave me one of the exaggerated kisses Alan had shown him.

"Mwah!" he said, grinning.

"Mwah yourself," I said. I put him down and he went back to his cards. I stood there for several minutes and let the feeling sink in. Miles was better. He still had a way to go, but my heart was finally at ease. The delays were present, but the roots of autistic behavior were gone, and I could project the normal development that was yet to come. I did not care how many people claimed it was impossible. Miles was going to recover from autism.

In the summer of 1996, Alan and I went to the second annual DAN! Conference, sponsored by Rimland's Autism Research Institute. The first DAN! Conference had not been open to the public. It was made up of twenty-eight handpicked scientists and physicians, and only four parents, including Lisa Lewis. At the second conference more parents were permitted to attend, and many of the physicians there were also parents of autistic children. Paul Shattock did not attend, but we would meet him shortly afterward when he came to give a talk at Alan's division of Johnson & Johnson.

Sidney Baker, a distinguished physician from Connecticut, had done a fine job of describing the theories of the autistic disease process and the many pieces of the puzzle. One notable speaker was Dr. Sudhir Gupta, who had successfully used immunoglobulin treatment to repair the damaged immune systems of a few children with autism, some of whom had shown dramatic improvement, and one of whom was reported to have had a complete recovery.

I said hello to Bill Shaw, the pathologist who had discovered the fungal metabolites (yeast waste products) in autistic urine, and whom I had once driven to the airport. He was speaking at the conference against the wishes of his former employer, the Children's Mercy Hospital of Kansas City. By going public with the information about yeast and fungus in autism, he was putting his career at risk, but he felt that the information was too important to keep to himself. He hoped that the many physicians in attendance at DAN! would find his piece of the puzzle useful in the treatment of their patients. As a result of his scheduled appearance, he had just been given notice, and was now unemployed.

Dr. Sinaiko was there, too, and I was happy to see him again. He had a wonderful smile and a quick intelligence, and I was reminded of Dr. Robinson and the pleasure it gave me to speak with a physician who was responsible yet open-minded. I introduced him to Alan, and we discussed testing for phenol sulfur transferase deficiency during a break in the sessions.

Alan understood the science behind the lectures, helping me to understand the practical outcome of each speaker's work. He shook his head after one environmental physician gave a talk about the data he had gathered on immune system abnormalities in autism. "This is not good science," he said. "This is not theory-driven science. I'm glad Susan Hyman isn't here—she'd be horrified."

"Yes, but, do you think they're right?" I asked.

"They might be," he admitted. "Yes, I think they probably are right, but medical science becomes accepted after following certain channels. If they don't follow these channels, no matter how true their findings are, they will be relegated to quackery. This is exactly what we *don't* want to happen."

CHAPTER FIVE

Red Flags

The most difficult and trying thing in my life was no longer fear about Miles's future, but the daily question of what he should eat. If someone had asked me when Miles was a baby if he had had food allergies, I would have said I did not think so. Now it appeared that he was allergic to almost everything.

We had made an interesting observation when we took Miles off soy. He had seemed fine while drinking soy milk every day, but when it was removed from his diet and reintroduced, he had an obvious allergic reaction. Just a trace of wheat-free soy sauce gave him hives and a severe diaper rash. After seeing this effect several times we were extremely careful to keep soy out of his diet.

Unfortunately, this phenomenon occurred with many other foods as well. It seemed to be true that the allergies were not apparent to us until the foods were removed and reintroduced. Miles's allergist, Dr. Park, told us he had seen this happen before. He explained that the allergy had probably been there, perhaps causing other problems, but that constant exposure to the food masked some of the symptoms. This, in general, is why allergy shots work. Small, consistent amounts of an allergen can reduce a reaction. In this case, however, the behavioral reaction was not being masked, only the physical one.

"Regular allergies are IgE-mediated, and I call them type I," he explained. "The allergies you describe are probably IgG-mediated, or what I call type II. We are only just beginning to see scientific evidence that such allergies really do exist."

What he recommended was called an "elimination diet," in which all common allergens were removed for a period of time, then reintroduced one at a time.

I was still confused about the two types of allergy, since IgE and IgG did not mean anything to me. Dr. Park explained that in the primary type, symptoms such as hives, swelling, or difficulty breathing were common reactions. I remembered that my nephew had such a problem with peanuts—my sister had to keep an epi-pen, an adrenaline shot, with him at all times.

In the secondary type of allergy, which must have been what we were seeing with Miles, a different part of the immune system seemed to be affected, and the response to such allergens could be headache, diarrhea, constipation, skin problems, irritability, disorientation, or even depression or hyperactivity. I was fascinated but a bit skeptical. Hyperactivity from food? I had skimmed through Doris Rapp's book *Is This Your Child?*, looking for references to cow's milk, and had seen some references to this, but it struck me as rather implausible.

The next time I visited the allergist's office, while waiting for the doctor, I chatted with one of the nurses on his staff. She nodded when I brought this up.

"I was trained by a doctor who would have laughed at any parent who said such a thing, but what I've seen since I've worked here has blown my mind. There are medical professionals who would rather stick to standard procedure than actually help their patients, but Dr. Park is not one of them."

"What kind of things have you seen here?" I asked.

"Well, we had one little boy in here who was the sweetest, calmest thing. He smiled at us and sat on Mom's lap. Then we were doing the skin testing, and after a provocation with corn—holy cow! In about two minutes that little boy went nuts, angry and screaming, knocking things over, slapping his mother again and again. He was just a different child. He's doing great now, no problems at school, lots of friends. He's scared to death of eating corn—says he doesn't like the way it makes him feel. His mom gets him maple candy from Canada instead of regular candy with corn syrup."

"I guess that's the kind of thing you have to see with your own eyes to believe," I said thoughtfully.

"All I know is, he would have been subjected to a lot of child psychology if his mom hadn't brought him here first—corn is in everything. And you know, that's not all. There was a teenage girl in here about five years ago on a ton of Prozac. She was up and down, well, mostly down and terribly depressed. Her mother was sure she was going to lose her. When we did the provocation testing with her, she was sitting here smiling and talking, and then when she got red food dye, she just curled up in the corner and said she wanted to die. In the fetal position—I'll never forget the sight of it."

"What happened?" I asked worriedly.

"Oh, she got the dyes and artificial flavors out of her diet and she did real well, real fast. She got right off the Prozac and went on with her life. We just got a card from her—she's in college. You bet I believe this stuff. I don't understand it, but I believe it."

Once again, I had a sinking feeling that I had been too smug in my skepticism about everything unproven. Well, maybe my skepticism was okay, but I was learning a very important lesson.

If something has been proven, it is probably true. If something has not been proven, it may or may not be true. *"Not proven" does not mean "false."*

Wow, what a concept that was for me to grasp. This should not have been so surprising, after my experiences with Miles, but it was then that my faith in medical protocol really began to crumble like a doughnut dipped in milk.

That night I asked Alan if he thought removing the dairy and then the wheat could have caused the other allergies to suddenly emerge. He thought about this for a moment.

"I think it's possible that his immune system was so swamped with the gluten and casein that when they were eliminated his system just attacked everything else that he ate. If it's true that the gut is leaky, then the foods might be going undigested into the bloodstream, which is triggering the unusual amount of reactivity. Too much of this could be partially responsible for the autistic symptoms."

"Like, they're living with a general discomfort level that is so high and causes so much interference that they become withdrawn?"

"Maybe. It might explain why Miles gets worse from corn, which doesn't yet seem to be linked to opiate activity."

There were still so many maybes. But one thing I was certain of was that Miles was not the only autistic child with multiple allergies. Because of my involvement in the community-wide effort to improve services for children with autism, I was meeting a lot of other parents. I got into the habit of asking them about what their children ate.

Almost universally, I heard the complaint that their children were very limited in the foods they would eat. But the foods were almost always the same foods: those containing dairy and/or wheat. The most commonly craved foods in almost all of these children were: milk, pizza, grilled cheese, macaroni and cheese, pasta, Cheerios, crackers, bread, and breaded chicken or fish—all foods composed of wheat and/or milk. A few of them liked tomatoes, apples, cocoa, and bananas, which were foods high in phenols and/or sugar. If Rosemary Waring, a British researcher, was correct, these were foods to be avoided as well. She had determined, by feeding a test group of autistic children acetaminophen and then later testing their urine, that many of them showed an impaired ability to break down the phenols in food.

The only food that they seemed to enjoy which did not fall into this category was french fries, and that made me wonder. Potatoes were one of the only things that Miles liked and could tolerate. Then I discovered that most brands of french fries were coated with wheat gluten to make them crispy and to keep them from sticking together. This does not need to be specified on the package label. Somehow, I had assumed that it was the manufacturer's job to inform me of what was in all of my food, but I was mistaken. When Burger King had decided to add gluten and whey to their fries, I had only found out because of the Internet.

Conversely, maybe some autistic people liked certain brands of fries because they *did not* affect them in any way. I had observed that some autistic children hated milk and dairy products, and their parents had to sneak dairy into their diets because they believed that such foods were necessary. Perhaps this was some kind of self-regulatory effect on the part of the children.

I once read about a study where a cat was given a new food that he had never tasted before—say, lamb. A few hours later he was given an emetic to induce vomiting. Weeks, months, even years later, that same cat would not eat lamb if it were presented to him. The memory of the illness was permanent. Lamb probably smelled like sickness to him. (I remember what happened to me in college the first time I drank peach schnapps, and the aversion I still have to the very smell of the stuff.)

It was interesting that my husband, Alan, hated the taste of bread. He had always avoided crackers, pretzels, cake, cookies, and anything containing wheat. It was reasonable to assume that, at a young age, Alan associated the taste of wheat with a bad feeling. That, and his parents' removal of dairy from his diet at his doctor's suggestion, might explain his "spontaneous recovery," or the fact that he had never really developed autism at all. Perhaps this was supported by the additional fact that he had not been given antibiotics for his ear infections, or vaccines, until he was much older than Miles. Three years earlier, after Miles's experience began, Alan had removed all gluten from his own diet and found that it was not a difficult change for him. He remains on a gluten-free diet; he believes it improves his digestion.

I remembered reading in *A Parent's Guide to Autism* that limited food choices were common. This was considered to be part of these children's desire for sameness. So why were they always the same type of foods? Why didn't I ever meet a parent whose autistic child craved popcorn, hamburgers, tuna fish, Twinkies, chocolate, or strawberries? Paul Shattock's theory made sense to me. If a child is getting a small amount of opiates from the improper breakdown of certain foods, he would begin to crave them. Every time the drugs wore off, he would go through withdrawal and feel terrible until he got more.

I suddenly pictured Miles standing in the living room, screaming inconsolably like a child with an unbearable headache, getting no relief until he drank a five-ounce bottle of milk. He would drink the entire thing at once. If we refilled it, he would again drink the entire thing. The only time I saw Miles leave over an ounce of milk was after drinking fourteen ounces.

Five ounces of milk, every hour. Sometimes every forty minutes. Up to seventy ounces a day. And no one thought anything was wrong with it. I felt like kicking myself. Every time I handed Miles a bottle of milk, I might as well have been handing him a bottle of lead paint.

Then, when we took dairy away, he began to crave pasta. Eating four or five servings at a sitting, shoveling it into his mouth as fast as he could, Miles had then become addicted to wheat. Perhaps it was not as good a "fix" for him as the dairy, but it was better than anything else he got.

Now that I was aware of his problem foods, Miles was doing so much better. Still, his diet was extremely limited. He was completely off dairy and gluten, and had noticeable reactions to corn, soy, egg yolk, tomato, fruits, vegetables, nuts, and legumes. I had some luck blending white root vegetables such as parsnips into his rice muffins, but mainly he ate potatoes, rice, and chicken. I gave him some liquid multivitamins twice each day, but I was still anxious about his nutrition.

Luckily, I was not alone. The many parents on the Internet with whom I had been corresponding had also described the identical pattern of food allergies. It amazed me that some of their children were reactive to the exact same foods that affected my son.

But I was not comfortable with giving my son a vegetable-free diet. In an effort to widen the variety of nutrients in Miles's food, I decided to puree and mix some yellow squash into his amaranth muffin batter. The muffins came out great, and he loved them. Even Laura had two. Then, several hours later, Miles began to cry. I put him on the changing table and was horrified to see a hot, red diaper rash. The next day his bottom was covered with bleeding fissures, cracked and sore. He sobbed as I wiped away the diarrhea, repeating pathetically, "No, pwease, don't, pwease wait . . . all done . . ."

This was inexcusable. I was in tears myself. My efforts at a varied diet would have to wait, at least until Miles was potty-trained.

Then one day, Alan met a visiting colleague at work who was allergic to everything but potatoes. Apparently, he lived on vitamins and potatoes and ate french fries at least once every day. He was in good health, and we were reassured. I asked Dr. Hyman about this, and she assured me that a child could probably develop very well on fried potatoes and chicken, with a good vitamin supplement that included iron. Miles's dairy substitute, the potato-based DariFree beverage, contained plenty of calcium. Meat and chicken contain all of the essential amino acids.

I suddenly realized that my desire to feed Miles a variety of foods was for my benefit more than his. Plain rice was the same as rice pasta, rice cakes, or pancakes made with rice flour. As long as he was happy and his blood tests showed no deficiencies, I could relax and change my standards for nutrition.

I wrote out a weekly diet for Miles (see Part Two, Chapter 12), and we stuck to it. In an effort to ensure that Miles would not develop an allergy to rice, we kept his diet rice-free three times a week. Wednesday was a potato-free day. I experimented with some gluten-free recipes and made him special pancakes, cookies, and muffins (see Part Two, Chapter 13). After some cautious trials with nuts and seeds, I made nut butter balls from ground sesame, sunflower, and macadamia nuts mixed with powdered DariFree and honey. After a few weeks the diet became easy to maintain.

DON'T DRINK YOUR MILK

I went to another autism conference, this time in Orlando. It was sponsored by the Feingold Association, the group that had been pioneering special diets for children with ADHD, attention deficit hyperactivity disorder, for decades. I sat in the back row, next to a parent named Portia Iversen.

I had been hoping to meet Portia. She and her husband, Jon Shestack, were founders of CAN, the Cure Autism Now foundation. CAN was predominantly a fundraising organization, raising money to fund research projects for which the National Institutes of Health had not allocated enough. Lisa Lewis, with whom I had often chatted on the phone, had spoken highly of her. In sorting through all of the hyperbole on the Internet, I had learned to trust Lisa's judgment.

Portia and Jon worked in Hollywood, and were shrewd, intelligent, and well connected. They put their knowledge of how to raise money to produce films and TV into CAN, and it flourished into a major fundraising entity.

In 1997, CAN started the AGRE (Autism Genetic Resource Exchange) project. Because scientists believed that three to five genes may be contributing to autism, they estimated that a minimum of one hundred families were needed to begin serious genetic linkage studies. The last research group to attempt this took over ten years and failed to share samples with other researchers. AGRE's first goal was to enroll a hundred families with more than one member affected by autism, PDD, or Asperger's syndrome, and to somehow do it within one year.

Initially, it looked like an impossible task, but with the help of Marianne Toedtman, the AGRE family coordinator, and thanks to a network of families and professionals across the country, the goal was actually exceeded. When the year had passed, there were over 450 families in the AGRE autism gene bank.

In January 1998, blood samples began to be taken from the "multiplex" families by experienced phlebotomists provided by CAN. In addition, a diagnostician was provided to assess the autistic individuals using the ADI (Autism Diagnostic Interview) test. By the fall of 1998, research samples were cataloged and available to the entire research community.

Portia was truly remarkable—she oversaw every step of the process, meeting with hundreds of consultants and insisting that the project be done properly. Special codes were developed to identify blood and samples without personal identifying information. This ensured privacy, and that no two researchers unknowingly utilized the same sample sets.

CAN then formed collaborative relationships with UCLA, the University of Washington, Mount Sinai Medical Center in Manhattan, Columbia University, the University of Chicago, and a European collaborative autism genetics group called P.A.R.I.S., to put the AGRE gene bank to its best use.

Portia also helped to put together the CAN Consensus Statement, a document that was created with input from over a hundred professionals. Its purpose was to provide parents, professionals, government support agencies, and insurance companies with a comprehensive guide to an appropriate, complete medical workup in autism.

In addition to being such an able crusader for research, Portia was a fine person. She had already met Alan at a conference in New York City, and after we discussed dietary intervention for a while, she asked if he and I were willing to participate in a CAN Parent Advisory Board. I gladly accepted her offer. Later, we went over the new NIH statistics.

"Four children out of every eighteen hundred," she said, "what does that come out to? And why do they put it like that?"

"I don't know, it's ridiculous," I replied. "Let's see—that makes one out of every . . . four hundred and fifty children. Can that be right? One in four-fifty?"

"Wow, that is high." Portia sighed. "That number has gone up in the past two years. And based on the paltry amount of funding it gets from the NIH, you'd think that it was a very rare disease."

"One in—my God. Portia, I felt like autism snuck into my house at night and stole my child's spirit, leaving only his body behind. If that many children were being physically kidnapped, we'd be in a state of national emergency."

She nodded silently, then murmured, "You're right. You're absolutely right. Hey, can I use that in our literature?"

I laughed.

The conference was fun. I met Dr. William Crook, who had written *The Yeast Connection.* Dr. Crook was very different from the way I had imagined him to be. I knew that much of the medical community had classified him as a crackpot for blaming behavioral disorders on a bunch of invisible, theoretical fungi in the digestive system, but although elderly, he was a lucid, intelligent man, a no-nonsense conventional physician with half a century of practical experience. With what I now suspected about candida and autism, I wondered whether time would vindicate his theories. He knew how many people he had helped, and was resolute in his belief that yeast and other sugar-eating bacteria were responsible for obesity, health problems, and behavioral problems in children and adults.

Kelly Dorfman, a nutritionist who was working with many autistic children, gave a talk on their special nutritional needs. I had a fascinating dinner with Jean Curtin (a parent I had met back home who was very knowledgeable about the diet), Bob Sinaiko, and Brenda O'Reilly from the AIA (Allergy Induced Autism) group in England, who had given a talk about the phenol sulfur transferase deficiency found in many autistic children.

I also heard a talk by Dr. William Cade, who was looking at urinary peptides in his lab at the University of Florida, with similar findings to those of Paul Shattock and Kalle Reichelt. He had originally discovered these substances in the urine of people with schizophrenia, and then later in those with autism. When his schizophrenic patients implemented the gluten-free, dairy-free diet, many of them experienced a spontaneous remission.

Just before the conference ended, I bought a paperback from the book table called *Don't Drink Your Milk* by Frank Oski, the former director of pediatrics at Johns Hopkins Medical School. In it he cited numerous reasons why dairy products were unsuitable foods for both children and adults. I was lactose intolerant, but took enzymes so that I could continue to eat dairy. The book convinced me to decide on a trial period without any dairy at all.

The more I read about milk, the more I wished mankind had never thought to drink a product from the udder of a cow. How absurd that seemed, now that I gave it some thought.

Humans evolved for thousands of years, weaned from their mother's milk by the age of three. Then suddenly, they continued the process of ingesting milk from another source—another species—because it was inexpensive, filling, and tasted good.

With a functional immune system, milk should be digestible. But what if environmental factors are altering children's immune systems so that milk is no longer beneficial, but harmful? A few months later I read that Dr. Oski had died, and felt a sense of loss.

I decided to take all dairy out of Laura's diet as well. She had no behavioral problems that I was aware of, but after reading about several studies linking milk to ear infections, sinus infections, and respiratory problems, I decided that there was no reason why she could not get her calcium from another source, such as the potato-based dairy substitute that Miles was using. Laura frequently asked for it instead of milk, and she ate plenty of protein. As far as I could tell, the only real health benefit from milk was calcium. The *only* one. And there were many other sources of that. How had the media made me think that it was the milk itself that was so important? It wasn't just the photos of celebrities with milk mustaches, it was the idea that giving a child milk was equivalent to good parenting.

When I got home, I talked to Laura about the experiment, and she didn't mind a bit. There did not seem to be any change in her behavior for the first few days, but something odd did happen. She was still suffering from night waking, which *stopped* immediately after she stopped drinking milk. No bad dreams, no crying out at night, nothing. For the last few months Laura had been up at least once each night crying and complaining that her room was shaking. When we asked what she meant, she merely sobbed, "It's shaking—my room is shaking."

Not conditioned by thirty years of milk drinking, Laura liked the milk substitute better than I did. But I learned to use it in my cereal, and enjoyed it in baked goods and homemade ice cream. I liked the fact that my stomach had lost its perpetually bloated feeling. Eight weeks later my motivation to use it grew even stronger.

At a friend's house, Laura and I both ate some pizza. It was all there was to eat—I had forgotten to mention the dairy restriction when we were invited for lunch. Just this once, I told her.

That night, Laura was up four times, after two months of not waking at all, up four times sobbing the once familiar phrase, "My room is shaking." As for me, my sinuses became blocked within half an hour. Then, a slow migraine began to creep up the back of my neck—the first one I'd had in months. Over the next year Laura on four occasions ate dairy by mistake, which coincided with exactly four episodes of night waking.

After having suffered from chronic sinus infections for most of my life, I realized that they had completely ceased. In fact, I was only sick once in an entire year—with a stomach flu that I caught at work. An entire winter miraculously passed without anyone in my family needing a course of antibiotics. Could this really be from removing the milk from our diets?

As much as I had loved pizza, as much as mixing up the fruit from the bottom of a cup of yogurt had been a religious experience for me, I did not want to eat dairy anymore. The very thought revolted me.

My headaches had truly stopped. My sinuses were clear.

However, my health had been unstable for several years, and I had believed my doctors when they told me that fatigue, pain, and frequent illness were normal in mothers of young children. Typically, I had brushed aside my petty maladies with annoyance, only succumbing to them a few times a year, when I simply could not get out of bed.

Now, after having been through the situation with Miles, I began to think about my own biggest complaints. I listed them on a piece of paper and realized that they resembled the symptoms of food allergy and yeast overgrowth:

- Extreme fatigue
- Disorientation and brain fog
- Diarrhea and bloating

Then I listed some of my lesser complaints:

- Joint pain and morning stiffness
- Always feeling cold
- Sleep disorder
- Intolerance to pain
- Difficulty exercising
- Sugar cravings
- Caffeine intolerance
- Back pain
- Frequent muscle spasms
- Clothes and shoes uncomfortable and restrictive

At twenty-three, I was diagnosed with CFS (chronic fatigue syndrome) after a virus that resembled hepatitis. After that, my energy seemed to have been permanently sapped. Ten years later I still woke up feeling exhausted.

After a chat with Bill Shaw, I decided to ask my gynecologist for a prescription for oral nystatin, and I carefully avoided all cookies, candy, fruit, and other sources of sugar that could aggravate a yeast problem.

The first two days were almost unbearable, as my craving for sugar reached new heights. I hung in there, imagining that I had a colony of parasites in my body, causing me to crave the only food that would keep them alive, regardless of its damage to my well-being. I was only half joking when I told Alan that I could knock a kid over in the street for a chocolate bar.

By the third day, the cravings had gone down. At the end of a week I found myself turning down a slice of birthday cake with genuine disinterest. After a month, my appetite had decreased, my clothes fit me better, and I felt healthier than I had in years. My other complaints remained, but my energy level and feeling of well-being increased noticeably.

I presented this information at the next meeting of the dietary support group I had started in my living room and that now included about twenty families. I was surprised to discover that a few of the mothers in the group had also responded well to an antiyeast program, and several had also been diagnosed with CFS at some point in their lives. There were twelve women at the meeting, and six of them had been diagnosed with something I had never heard of—fibromyalgia syndrome. They explained that FMS was characterized by chronic fatigue and pain. It had been theorized that it was the second stage of CFS rather than a separate disease.

"Doesn't this seem like a bit of coincidence?" I asked. "That fifty percent of this group has fibromyalgia?"

Kathy Terrillion laughed. "Not really," she said. "FMS is probably an immune system disorder. The predisposition to it is probably genetic. Our kids must have the same predisposition, but in their cases it just combined with other factors to manifest as autism."

"Wait, I just had a thought," I said excitedly. "What if the age of onset determines the ultimate diagnosis? Like, if a whole family has the predisposition, some kind of 'global immune dysfunction syndrome,' and a virus or something is the trigger, then a one-year-old ends up with autism, a seven-year-old gets ADHD, and an adult gets chronic fatigue?"

There were murmurs of assent, and then I amended my thought. "On the other hand, I may be oversimplifying. I think that the autistic kids are being *much* further impaired by the problem. Maybe autism is the ultimate disease state. Like, if whatever caused autism happened to an adult, they would probably get . . ." I thought hard for a moment, and then was struck by the answer. *"Schizophrenia."*

"Which is the disorder that Dr. Cade was studying when he first found the urinary gluten and casein peptides," Kathy added, following my thoughts.

I was raised by my mother, and had little contact with my father's children until I was an adult, but I was aware that I had had an older half-sister on my father's side whom my family rarely spoke about named Jennifer. She had been a timid, highly sensitive soul, often in her own world. "Vulnerable" was the word that was often used to describe her. She had been diagnosed with juvenile schizophrenia, and had jumped out of a window in 1974, when I was nine. I wasn't told until years later. Another of my half-siblings on that side was a brother, Jonathan, who had been institutionalized as a child for what appears to have been rage, impulsivity, and aggression. I never met him. As far as I knew, he was still in a state institution. Yet another, as an adult, suffers from episodes of psychosis. Two more of my father's children are highly intelligent, functional adults, both of whom are now physicians.

I'd always thought my family was fairly typical, but after Miles was diagnosed and we saw a geneticist, I began to discover that there were a surprising number of neurological and psychological disorders in both sides of my family as well, disorders commonly seen in the extended families of children with autism. In the geneticist's words, "There are a lot of red flags here."

I imagine that members of one family with a genetic predisposition toward immune dysfunction could share a disease that manifests in many different ways. How sad, and how strange, to wonder what would have happened to Jennifer and Jonathan if their own mother hadn't died young, or if they had lived thirty years later and had been children of mine.

It seemed that I had been spared any serious functional disorders, but I decided that I would talk to my new doctor about the pain and fatigue that seemed to be worse than ever. I had recently asked to be tested for rheumatoid arthritis, since the amount of pain I experienced in the morning was almost crippling, but the test results were negative. In caring for Miles, I admitted to myself that I had probably neglected my own health, and I decided to follow up. Sure enough, my symptoms matched those of fibromyalgia, and I discovered that the many sensitive spots on my body were called "tender points"—another criterion for diagnosis with FMS.

Researching the disorder on the Internet, I discovered exactly what I had suspected I would. Like autism, the disease was genetically predisposed. It was thought to be triggered by an insult to the immune system such as extreme stress, injury, or virus. I knew that the term "autoimmune" was being overused for modern illnesses, but it was suspected that fibromyalgia fell into that category. Many FMS sufferers controlled their illness with a combination of moderate exercise, yeast control, and allergy elimination diets. Oddly enough, suspect foods included the nightshades that my mother avoided because they gave her "arthritis": tomatoes, potatoes, peppers, and eggplant.

Dutifully, I eliminated those foods, which were among my favorites, and found immediate relief from my pain and stiffness. I consented to a prescription drug that helped me sleep more soundly and regularly. As a result of those two factors, for the first time in my adult life, I maintained an exercise program without missing a day. I discovered that eggs, oranges, and coffee had been causing my stomach problems. I took supplements of glucosamine, which also seemed to help control the joint pain.

Maintaining a low-sugar diet was important, too. When I was having a bad day of pain and fatigue, I usually found myself craving sugar to an almost unbearable extent, and it took great willpower to stay away from it. But now I knew what it felt like to feel good, and there was no going back. Although I still had some difficult days, for the most part I was well.

My house became cleaner, my office more organized, my thoughts less foggy, and my current relationship with my husband and daughter came sharply into focus. The tornado had blown through, and now it was cleanup time. I began making lists of things to do, instead of obsessing about how behind I was. I planned one-on-one time with

Laura and made myself slow down enough to enjoy it. The exercise was time-consuming, but left me more clearheaded. I was able to accomplish more in a day and knew when to quit.

"You know, you look great," Alan said one day as I got ready for bed. "You look like a model." I laughed. I had always complained of being ten pounds overweight. Then I looked in the mirror critically and realized that I had gone down a size. My waist was slimmer and less bloated. My skin looked healthy, and I appeared younger somehow. The difference was striking. The only thing that remained the same was the worried look in my eyes, the eyes of someone who knew too much. But the rest of me was in better shape than it had been in my entire adult life. The monster had invaded my home but had brought its own gifts. And I no longer believed in symptoms without cause.

CHAPTER SIX

"Trials"

One supplement that really seemed to help Miles was DMG, short for dimethylglycine. When we had first started giving him one tablet per day, he began putting two words together almost immediately. "Arm stuck" were his exact, appropriately used words. He also seemed clearer and more tuned in, as if a fog had been lifted from his brain.

I could not swear that there was a correlation, however. We had been traveling at that time, and my kids always seemed to have developmental growth spurts when we traveled.

Then, when we decided to try increasing Miles's DMG dosage, we did not tell Jill or Valerie, his speech therapist. Within two days we were surprised to hear from both of them regarding the improvement in his language. He was suddenly putting three- and four-word sentences together.

Valerie's notes read:

Miles was *highly* verbal today and had a great deal of spontaneous language. He was also quite silly—tickling me throughout the ses-

sion! More initiation on his part today and more verbal comment-
ing noted. *Good* eye contact.

We waited three weeks, then tried the same experiment. Jill phoned
me two days later. "Well, whatever you're doing, keep it up. I see a dramatic change in Miles again this week."
This is what Valerie wrote in her notes that day:

What a super session today! Miles made tremendous eye contact
today without cueing. Great expansion of spontaneous utterances,
also some five- to six-word utterances noted. Miles is also doing
better with use of sounds within words.

We still could not swear that these events were related to the DMG,
but as far as we knew the supplement was harmless. We believed we
had seen enough of a change to keep three tablets of DMG in Miles's
daily diet (see Part Two, Chapter 10, for more about DMG). Once
again, it came down to trusting our instincts; and balancing cost, limited studies, anecdotal evidence, and suspected improvement.

I began adding essential fatty acids, EFAs, to Miles's nut butter
balls in the form of flaxseed oil. EFAs were thought to improve brain
function, among other things, and after reading about the potential
benefits and reasons for deficiency, I decided that they were something
we should all be taking. I also began supplementing Miles with extra
vitamin C (not megadoses, just a couple of extra chewables each day),
in addition to his multivitamin.

I got a flyer in the mail from Bill Shaw. He had started his own
reference lab, the Great Plains Laboratory, in Overland Park, Kansas.
From there he was doing the urine testing for fungal metabolites ("yeast
poop," as my friends and I called it) that indicated a need for antifungal
treatment. I was glad to hear from him. After his courage in attending
the DAN! Conference, I believed that he deserved great success.

Unfortunately, the news from Bob Sinaiko was not as good. One of his patients, a little boy with ADHD, was being successfully treated with nystatin and dietary intervention. The child's mother had brought him to Dr. Sinaiko and was pleased with the results. However, the child was the subject of a custody battle, and the father cited the use of this "quack therapy" to strengthen his case. The case was brought before the California Board of Medicine, and Bob's medical license was in jeopardy. Even though the treatments he had advocated were safe, they deviated from standard medical practice.

. Dr. Sinaiko's patients rose up in arms and established a legal defense fund. Parents of autistic children everywhere grew alarmed, and saw this as a terrible threat to the freedom of their physicians to help them help their children. The battle over Dr. Sinaiko's right to practice medicine wages on in California, where I believe that much more is at stake than the mere livelihood of a superb physician and a thoroughly decent human being.

Alan was working as a scientific researcher for Ortho, a division of Johnson & Johnson that developed clinical diagnostics. At his request he was given approval to begin a side project looking for a marker for autistic kids that could someday be used as a routine neonatal or postnatal diagnostic test to indicate an appropriate treatment. He began by setting up a test to look for the neuropeptides that had been identified by Shattock and Reichelt, to see if he could confirm that they really were casomorphin and alpha-gliadin, as well as to look for any other unusual substances.

Meanwhile, I was doing some research of my own. I knew about a dozen sets of parents who were doing a home-based behavioral program with their autistic children. I had spoken to them a few times about trying the diet. Most were skeptical, and many felt that they simply could not do any more than they were already doing. The discrete trial program was taxing, especially for those who were trying to maintain up to forty hours of therapy per week for their children. At first only six of the mothers were willing to try the diet.

Two of the boys craved milk and drank it to excess. They had chronic diarrhea and a history of antibiotic use and red cheeks. They, like Miles, responded well to having dairy removed from their diets. Both had formed bowel movements for the first time in months with the removal of gluten. All began to show allergic reactions to other foods, such as soy, corn, and egg yolk. At first I dubbed them the "Gluten Kids."

Two other children, both female, were very different. Both Chelsea and Larisa ate a lot of bread and cheese, but were notable for craving foods high in phenols, such as bananas, peanut butter, and apples. Their bowel movements were only mildly abnormal, and they did not have much of a history of ear infections and antibiotics, although both were susceptible to yeast infections. Their reaction was less obvious.

When put on an elimination diet the "Phenol Kids" surprised their parents by getting bright pink cheeks when phenolic foods were reintroduced. Chelsea, for the first time in her life, opened the cupboard and climbed up the shelves, looking for the foods she was being denied. She had her first real tantrum when she pulled at the milk carton and was refused. Her mother's solution was to pour some rice milk into a clean milk carton before serving it.

At first Chelsea clearly showed some improvement, but not nearly to the same extent that Miles did. Since her initial response to the diet was not particularly dramatic, I assumed that she would not be a responder. Over the next few years, however, Chelsea was to do remarkably well. When she started the diet, she had been undersized and sickly, but her parents did extensive testing and, with the help of Kelly Dorfman, the nutritionist who saw a lot of autistic patients, put her on a vitamin supplementation program that enabled her to grow into a tall, healthy, able little girl. After three years on the diet her autism faded so significantly that she began the first grade without supports, receiving only speech therapy once a week.

Meanwhile, Lori, Larisa's mother, told me that she saw an improvement in the first few weeks but had trouble attributing it to diet. Then, when she introduced the first phenolic food (bananas) into Larisa's diet, the little girl's cheeks became pink and she stayed up until late at night, laughing maniacally in her crib. Lori then realized that this nighttime laughing had been absent, and she hadn't even noticed it. A second trial a week later brought her again to this conclusion. She sent me an e-mail headed, "Yes, We Have No Bananas!"

Lori and I had become friends, and at times our friendship was a poignant one. In the story of the Pied Piper, one little boy did not make it into the mountain on time and was the only child returned to his family. Long ago, hearing this story, I had imagined the feelings of his mother, desperately glad to have her child back but forever having to contend with the sorrow of the others.

I thought about Larisa frequently. What were we missing? Since Miles's problem seemed to be that he could not break down certain proteins, removing the proteins had done the trick. Larisa was already off casein and gluten. I suggested removing soy, which seemed to make only a very slight difference, if any.

One parent impressed me with the alacrity with which she agreed to try the diet. Terri Kerr had two boys, both with a PDD diagnosis. I had come to realize that pervasive developmental disorder, although slightly differently defined in the *DSM* (*Diagnostic and Statistical Manual of Mental Disorders*), was often a doctor's way of *not* diagnosing autism. Several children I knew had been diagnosed with "high-functioning PDD." When I met them, they seemed to be clearly autistic. I discovered that one of the physicians in my area preferred it because "it was easier on the parents not to have to deal with the label of autism." In many cases this also meant that the child qualified for fewer hours of educational services.

Anyway, Terri Kerr knew that what her boys had *was* autism, and she left no stone unturned to find out what she could do to help. Perhaps one of the reasons she acted so swiftly was her own health. Terri was a young, beautiful woman with a serious heart condition whose doctor had told her that her life expectancy was uncertain. She was willing to try the diet for the boys within a few minutes of speaking with me on the phone.

"I believe it was the MMR vaccine that started their problems," she told me.

I replied politely. "Yes, I've heard people say that before. The vaccine does coincide with the typical age of onset."

"Well, in the case of my boys, it coincided pretty dramatically. Ian was completely normal until that day. Kyle was hospitalized later that week, and was never the same."

Ian, the older boy, was fairly high-functioning when he began the diet at six. He responded dramatically, gaining language rapidly and catching up with his peers within months. He would later achieve normal functioning, with a learning disability but little or no residual traces of autism. Kyle was a different story, gaining some social skills and experiencing moderate improvement, but achieving little useful language. For him, the disease seemed to have hit much harder.

Two brothers, each with a different response to the diet. Although I had broken the children into subgroups, I really felt that they were suffering from the same underlying cause, but I just didn't know what that was. Removing dairy and gluten made a huge difference for Lisa Lewis's son, Sam, but Sam was still being affected by something. Larisa had been off of the foods for ages, and she was still autistic. Something was still there. What was it?

Some researchers, like William Shaw, seemed to think that much of the immune problem of people with autism begins when candida is not destroyed before turning into its mycelial form. This fungal form of candida, besides being invasive, had certainly been implicated in a variety of disorders in Dr. Crook's *Yeast Connection*. I remembered from the Feingold Conference that Crook also attributed such things as depression, chronic fatigue, and obesity to the overgrowth of mycelial candida.

I felt a surge of desperate hope. What if it were all as simple as preventing the overgrowth of candida? We had not attributed much of Miles's success to the nystatin, and had not even understood at first why we were giving it to him. Perhaps it *had* played an important role in his success. Perhaps it was doing something besides killing candida, something that helped reduce the number of neuropeptides that were being produced.

It had been suggested that in some individuals candidiasis occurs because of an immune defect. In others, it may occur because of their overuse of antibiotics. What if Larisa was in the former group and Miles in the latter, and his later onset of the problem made him respond more readily? Lisa Lewis had told me that Sam had been tested and briefly treated for yeast, but that it didn't seem to be a problem for him.

I called Lori and asked her if Larisa was taking nystatin. I knew a lot of the kids were, and I was excited to hear that she was not. Lori had tried many other things, like B vitamins and DMG. In fact, she had been the one who had recommended that we begin using DMG. She had missed Shaw's talk at the conference, and I summarized the theory of gastrointestinal yeast overgrowth.

"Did you see a difference in Miles when you started the nystatin?"

"Well, he seemed a lot less drunk, and stopped staggering around. At first I thought it was the removal of gluten, which we tried at the same time. But I've heard other parents say that the drunken behavior in their kids stopped with the antifungals, so now I suppose that could be what did it."

"Well, Larisa does that lurching walk. I'll ask the doctor for a prescription for nystatin. It couldn't hurt to try."

I waited eagerly for an e-mail. Lori and I did not have much time to gab on the phone, so we stayed in touch with little computer notes.

Karyn—Do you think nystatin could have gluten in it? Since she started it, Larisa has been having diarrhea and she's vomited four times. She is really cranky—worse than when we did the elimination diet. I think she's having a reaction to it. I'm going to stop giving it to her.

Could her bottle of nystatin be different than mine? If it contained gluten, I was sure Miles would have reacted to it. We compared notes on the telephone.

"Does it look like phlegm?" I asked.

"Yup. And it smells like cough syrup."

"That's the stuff. Amazing that I can slip it into his cup."

"Mmm. Maybe I can get it in a powdered form."

A few days later I phoned Jean Curtin, the local acquaintance who had been to the Feingold Conference. Jean's son, Michael, was a very bright nine-year-old whose autism had been brought to a fragile but admirable standstill using this biological approach. He was doing well in a regular school and had amazed his doctors with his transition from a seriously disabled, sickly, autistic four-year-old to a fairly healthy boy with only mild social differences.

Jean had been learning about this condition a lot longer than I had, and she had implemented the diet with Michael years before Miles was diagnosed. I had a lot of respect for what she had accomplished. Knowing more about autism than I once had, I could see that she was a person who was caring, bright, and insightful, but I wondered if most physicians would see much more than an eccentric parent. Perhaps this was how they saw me.

I asked Jean about Larisa, and described her maniacal laughing after eating bananas.

"In my experience, maniacal laughing and nighttime laughing have *always* been connected with a yeast problem, especially after eating sweet foods like bananas or sugar. Is she on an antifungal?"

"Well, she had a reaction to the nystatin. We were wondering if there might be gluten in her brand."

"No, not gluten. Let me guess, yeast was pouring out of every orifice? Diarrhea? Vomiting?"

"Yes! We thought it was a bad reaction."

"No, it sounds like she was having a massive die-off. I've seen it; it's revolting. When it happened to Michael, yeast was even pouring out of his nose."

"Holy cow. I guess Shaw had said something about a die-off, but it didn't sink in. Actually, Lori said the diarrhea looked like it was 'full of yeast.' I didn't even know what she meant when she said it. What should I tell her to do? Resume the nystatin?"

"She needs to be careful. I've heard of kids' lungs filling up with yeast. She should start with a really low dose, like half a mil every two days, than gradually work up to two mils. She should also be putting Lotrimin on any diaper rash."

I couldn't wait to tell Lori. That night I dreamed that Larisa began to talk.

Lori was apprehensive about resuming the liquid nystatin, but she was able to obtain some in its powdered form. This time Larisa's reaction was less dramatic, but the die-off did continue for several weeks. It was a month before I saw her again, and I was impressed by the change.

She was a lot less stimmy and spaced out. She really seemed to be looking at my children, and her vocalizations had increased. In addition, she had begun to cry when she fell down or hurt herself—something she had never done before. Lori's husband, Steve, who had been skeptical about the diet, was now convinced that there was a connection between it and the change in his daughter. Especially when Larisa began to use a few words, saying "hi" and "bye-bye" appropriately. However, her autism persisted. She was still removed from us by that indefinable, impenetrable wall.

How much could Larisa improve? She was only two and a half, but my suspicion was that she had a longer way to go than Miles. His entire decline had lasted only a few months, whereas Larisa had been different from birth—she was always easygoing and detached, and never reached the expected social developmental milestones. Or perhaps she had this disorder in a different form than Miles did and would never be able to recover fully.

If you put a patch over a newborn kitten's eye, after three weeks the eye will be functionally blind. Certain neurons are set up to be responsible for certain functions at certain critical times.

So to what extent could "metabolic brain damage" be reversed? I didn't know, but I knew from Terry Hines's classes that the preadolescent brain had a lot of plasticity, which meant that if one area of the brain was atrophied or damaged, other areas of the brain were able to take over its functions. I believed it was true for Miles. I had to hope that this would be the case for some of the others, too.

One little boy did not seem to have much in common with Miles. Bryan was very active and did not suffer from postural insecurity. At three and a half he was nonverbal but was showing signs of hyperlexia, an early ability to read. He was a placid, happy child who never cried. He did not have a history of antibiotic use, yeast infections, or food allergies. He did seem to enjoy a lot of phenolic foods, especially bananas.

The only similarity between Miles and Bryan was that Bryan had a lot of soft bowel movements—usually six or seven each day. Bryan really resembled Larisa more, which made me suspect that he would not respond the way that Miles did to the diet.

In the first week, Bryan's parents removed all dairy and gluten from his diet. Within twenty-four hours Bryan responded by having a formed bowel movement—and continued to do so once each day from then on. His disposition and ability to interact with others improved, and he willingly accepted new foods into his diet in that first week.

After the first week, Bryan began taking the antifungal nystatin. The first day or two after that were pretty bad, with tantrums, rubbing his head, and throwing himself on the floor. He even ran a low fever for a few hours. His therapists noted in his program notes that his behavior had greatly worsened.

"Could this be a virus?" I asked Angela, his mother. "It's possible that it's a coincidence."

"Bryan has *never* been sick before. This is the first time he's run a fever in his life. I find it hard to believe it's not due to the nystatin."

"Well, if so, then what I've heard is that this is a good sign—it's called a die-off reaction. That's what happened to Larisa. She was even vomiting. If Bryan did have gastrointestinal candidiasis, then killing the little beasties off might cause them to release toxins into his body. Check with your doctor, but I'd reduce the dose a little and maybe wait it out."

I hoped I knew what I was doing. Playing doctor with another person's child was a dangerous business. For the first time it occurred to me that I could actually be doing Bryan some harm. I was not recommending harmful drugs or inhumane aversives. Only nystatin, which battles yeast and fungus locally, in the gut. Still, I waited anxiously to hear from Angela. Two days later I got a phone call. Bryan had woken up a different child.

He was alert, cheerful, and started babbling—the same kind of babbling that we had heard from Miles when we first started the diet. Angela's voice was trembling with excitement.

"The change in him is really something," she said. "He is more aware of us than he's ever been. I cannot thank you enough."

I almost wished she had not thanked me—it made me feel a little bit embarrassed, and I still felt guilty for tampering with her son's health without really knowing what I was doing. Just hearing that Bryan had improved was such an overwhelming relief. That same day Angela phoned me again. Bryan had astonished his parents and therapists by making enormous gains in his therapy sessions, and topped it off with another surprise. He took five magnetic letters out of a box and put them on the refrigerator, carefully spelling out a word: B-R-Y-A-N.

Angela kept his diet very pure for ten more days. He ate white fish simmered in lemon juice, french fries cooked in canola oil, rice, chicken, and mashed potatoes with salt and olive oil. His improvement was remarkable. Then she decided to introduce a new food. She telephoned me early the next morning.

"We were up *all night* with Bryan. He was a mess, screaming, banging his head, hitting us and himself. It was the worst experience I've ever had with him. I never should have introduced a new food at night."

"What did you give him?"

"Get this—*half of a banana*. Three weeks ago they were his favorite food. Now I can see what they've been doing to his body and brain all this time."

"Bananas! That's what set Larisa off. She was up all night laughing maniacally. Bananas are very high in phenols—and sugar."

"Wow. Well, Bryan sure wasn't laughing."

"The poor little guy. It makes me wonder if that's what Miles was going through, maybe having terrible headaches. All that time that he spent screaming."

"It's so strange," said Angela. "Whatever it is, it has to make it hard for them to learn."

"I think if they are getting the foods every day, they get a certain level of 'white noise,' or 'interference,' that makes it difficult to deal with the world. When you take the foods away and reintroduce them, you can really see the reaction."

So perhaps phenols and yeast problems went hand in hand. Gluten, casein, a self-limited diet, and allergy seemed to go together. There was plenty of overlap between the groups. It was a very complicated puzzle. There was still something that I was missing, and I was confused.

I went to another conference, this time sponsored by the Westchester County (New York) Autism Society. Dr. Sidney Baker, from the DAN! group, was there, giving a lucid presentation on what was known so far about the biological causation of autism. I sat with Paul Shattock, who had become a friend, and absently jotted down notes about the findings of the different speakers.

Then Dr. John Martin spoke about a "stealth" virus he had found in the blood of autistic children, as well as in the blood of other dysfunctional individuals. I listened carefully, wondering if this accounted for one of the "immune insults" that I believed triggered the onset of the disorder.

He cited proof that the monkeys used in this country to culture human vaccines almost all test positive for simian cytomegalovirus (CMV), which is the monkey version of human cytomegalovirus. This is considered to be a harmless medium for culture, as the virus is unlikely to cross the species barrier.

However, he had found a virus in human subjects with various functional difficulties like chronic fatigue syndrome and Gulf War syndrome, and had traced it to a combination of simian cytomegalovirus and polio vaccine, along with other human viruses that had combined with a nasty result—a stealth virus that had tagged along on a vaccination and wreaked havoc on the immune system of its human host.

After the conference, Alan and I went out to dinner with John

Martin and Paul Shattock, and Alan Broughton from Immunoassay Labs, and we mulled it all over. It was a good meal. I was still uncertain about which pieces fit where, but we were on the right track, I just knew it.

The vague shape of the monster could be seen through the mist.

At about that time, Dr. Jeff Kopelson from Brewster, New York, phoned me to say that many of his patients' parents wanted to try the diet but were at a loss as to how to go about it. It was easy enough for him to tell them to take their children off of dairy and gluten, but difficult for them to do so without any good resources.

It was encouraging to hear that he recommended the diet for his autistic patients. One parent I knew told me that her pediatrician absolutely would not support her proposal that a gluten-free diet might help her son, since the child frequently suffered from constipation and probably needed *more* fiber in his diet. The doctor then ordered the blood test for celiac disease to prove his point, and astonishingly the test results came back positive!

I envied this child's parents, because now they were justified in doing the diet with full medical support. Most of the autistic children I knew who had the blood test did *not* have a positive result, although many were later diagnosed with CD based on the results of a small-bowel biopsy. I wished once again that I had insisted on a biopsy for Miles while he was still eating gluten, back when the results might have been positive.

Susan Hyman was not going so far as to recommend the diet outright, but she did mention it to a few parents at the point of diagnosis. One of her patients, a little boy who was under two and who craved milk, seemed to fit Miles's profile, and his mother, Lori Ross, agreed to give me a call. She was a nurse and her husband was a doctor, so they were reasonably skeptical, but still willing to give it a try.

Happily, Bobby's response was as immediate and dramatic as Miles's had been. He even developed almost the same pattern of food allergies that resulted in diarrhea.

I recommended Jill Pavone as Bobby's special-ed teacher, and she commented often on the similarities between the two boys. Although Bobby was a year younger than Miles, he started the diet at about the same age, and every time I saw him, I marveled at the likeness. Although he looked different, and certainly had developed a different personality, his progress over the next two years matched Miles's in an uncanny way. Seeing him always reminded me of what Miles had been doing and saying a year earlier.

This was a step toward convincing Susan Hyman that other patients of hers might benefit from the diet, although I knew she would not actually endorse it until it was medically accepted. Many more parents of her patients did call me after that, wanting the same kind of help that Dr. Kopelson's patients sought, and asking for my time.

I wished that Lisa Lewis's book had been published. She had explained to me that she was working on a comprehensive how-to for dietary intervention called *Special Diets for Special Kids*. I imagined how wonderful it would be if Dr. Kopelson could just tell his patients to buy the book, but the publication date was months away.

In the meantime, I agreed to visit his office and go over the nuts and bolts of the diet with several of his families, based on the individual problems and requirements of each child. Brewster was a six-hour drive from my house, but my sister lived nearby, and I could visit her for a couple of days.

When I arrived at his office, Jeff Kopelson and his staff set me up in an examining room. He had already reviewed his patients' test results with them, and had proposed a treatment plan. My job was to explain the diet, and one by one I described to different sets of parents what it was and how to get their kids to eat gluten-free foods. I reassured them that this was a worthwhile intervention to try, by explaining about

Miles and how well he had done, and gave them food suggestions that would substitute well for their children's favorites.

I was careful not to make any medical judgments or to give specific recommendations about vitamins and supplementation, since I was not a certified nutritionist, and that was the doctor's department. But I did explain that my son's diet was very limited, and that he was in good health with appropriate supplementation. I was surprised at how much I had learned from the numerous families in my area, and how many questions I was able to answer.

Many of the patients I saw were already doing an antifungal regimen, and several were already dairy-free. Although a few of their parents complained to me about the cost of the testing, most were excited and pleased with the results. While one patient's mother was disgruntled about her overall experience, the next could not praise Dr. Kopelson enough for how much he had helped her family. I decided that, as in everything else, a person has to make decisions about what medical course to pursue based on his or her own experience and judgment.

Dr. Kopelson was willing to go a step further than other physicians, and for that, most of his patients were grateful. Many had previously seen over twenty other doctors, and were only now getting some relief from the host of modern illnesses like fatigue, obesity, attention deficit, and autism. In some cases, the relief was dramatic. Most of the parents I saw had autistic children, but one or two others stood out in my mind because they seemed to be in the same immune system dysfunction category.

Dr. Kopelson was routinely sending blood from patients with mental dysfunction out to John Martin, and many of the samples tested positive for stealth virus. I had even sent a sample of my own blood, which came back negative. I was surprised, but glad in a way, to know that not every sample sent had a positive culture for the virus.

Jeff was excited about the fact that he was usually able to predict, with some accuracy, which patients' samples would test positive for stealth. Most of his patients with autism did test positive, as well as others with chronic fatigue syndrome and other mental dysfunctions.

For example, he had a patient, an older teenager, who was so badly afflicted by CFS that he could barely function. He had difficulty thinking or speaking clearly, and school had become impossible. His mother had to drive him to the office for the consultation. The onset had occurred about two years earlier, after what seemed to be a case of the flu.

Surprisingly, the boy's workup had revealed that his immune system was functioning very much like that of a child with autism. He tested positive for food allergies, candidiasis, abnormal immunoglobulin, and stealth virus. This made me think of my speculation about late-onset autism, and I wondered if this was some variation on the theme.

He was more of a man than a boy, tall, with rugged good looks, and probably once very popular with his high school friends. He could barely mumble a reply to my questions, and had to lie down on the exam table while I explained to his mother about a multiple-food elimination diet. She told me that every other doctor they had seen had said that there was nothing that could be done. Despite his protests, it had previously been recommended that he be treated for depression. I had a hopeful feeling that they were now on the right track.

Another nonautistic patient that I saw really surprised me. Dr. Kopelson asked me to step into his office and look at some results on the food allergy testing.

The testing that was then available for identifying what Dr. Park had called type II, or IgG, food allergies seemed to me to be unreliable. A sample of blood was used to determine a reactive response to over a hundred different foods, with results given as scores from 0.100 up. Foods with values under 0.200 were considered tolerable. After speaking to several people about foods that they knew to be a problem, and comparing them with these test results, I decided that any food with a value under 0.150 was probably safe, any food with a value over 0.250 was probably to be avoided, with the foods in the middle as a gray area to be determined by trial and error.

Among the autistic patients I often saw low values, such as 0.130, for foods that I considered to be low-risk, like celery, bean sprouts, ginger, honey, and lemon juice. Values for dairy and wheat products were consistently high, sometimes over 0.300. Most patients with autism seemed to have about a dozen foods besides dairy and gluten that were problematic.

I sat down in Dr. Kopelson's office, and he handed me a sheet of results.

"What do you make of that?" he asked.

I let out a low whistle. "Wow. This is amazing. I have never seen values like these before! . . . 0.574, wait, here's one at 0.622. This is incredible. There are at least thirty foods like this. Does this child have autism?"

"No . . . Down's syndrome."

I couldn't believe my ears. Everyone knew that Down's was caused by an extra chromosome in the twenty-first pair of chromosomes in their DNA.

"Down's syndrome? That seems impossible. I thought Down's was purely genetic."

"Well, yes, the occurrence is genetic. But the disease may be immunological, and treatable, to some degree. In this patient, at least, I believe that there is something that I can do to help."

A few minutes later I met the little boy and his mother, and observed that although the child was verbal and was actually doing quite well, he showed some overt signs of allergy, like itchy skin and dark circles under his eyes. His mother had long suspected that some foods made it harder for him to function and was willing to try restricting his diet. She told me that after speaking with a friend whose Down's child had been helped with vitamins and diet she had decided to give it a try. Dr. Kopelson had recently put her son on a vitamin supplementation program that seemed to be helping.

Whether this particular child's immune problems were coincidental to his Down's syndrome or whether the two were related was unclear. Dr. Rimland later sent me a videotape about the late Dr. Henry Turkel, who put Down's children on megadoses of multivitamins and found that the musculoskeletal and other outward features of the disease improved as much as did the subjects' mental functioning. If this was true, did it mean that there was some critical metabolic dysfunction and that early treatment could mean a reversal of symptoms? I just didn't have enough information to judge. But I did know that if I had a child with Down's, and the treatment appeared safe, I would certainly explore such a path.

The modern world becomes a lot less civilized when one realizes that we do not, in fact, know everything. The Romans probably thought that technology could not get much more advanced than their irrigation system. They had flushing toilets, for heaven's sake, and we think of them as uncivilized. When I read modern medical journals, I am frequently amazed at the time and money that is wasted on studies to determine things like whether breast-fed infants grow up to be better athletes, or whether sleep deprivation affects your ability to drive a car. Some results don't matter, some are obvious, and most won't affect our behavior or a treatment decision.

Just before Miles turned three, our school district set up his CPSE (Committee on Preschool Special Education) meeting. Jill, his special-ed teacher; Valerie, his speech therapist; and his schoolteachers had warned me that he was not going to meet the criteria for special-ed services.

How could that be? Didn't a diagnosis of autism in itself necessitate services? I had mixed feelings. On one hand, I knew that Miles was going to get better. He was already such a delight, and he was learning so fast that, although he was so young, Jill had nowhere to go in the Lovaas program but to move on to letter recognition, writing, and early reading skills. On the other hand, pulling the supports out from under him might result in a loss of momentum, or worse, a decline.

When I spoke with Dr. Hyman about this, she was disturbed. She did an informal exam and determined that there were still mild autistic abnormalities in Miles's behavior. His eye contact was inconsistent, his voice still lilted with an odd prosody, and his language was impressively rich and complex, but still somewhat stereotypical. She wrote a letter explaining that Miles still needed educational supports.

I let her write the letter, and I knew she believed that it was true. But deep down I wondered if she was mistaken. I liked and trusted Dr. Hyman very much, and I was trying to be fair, but it was hard to determine if we both truly lacked objectivity. I wanted to believe that Miles was better and that autism was treatable, and she wanted to uphold the credibility of her original diagnosis and the widely held belief that autism was incurable.

The school district was not going to be impartial either. They were bound by strict guidelines that determined what percentage of delay warranted special services, and they had a budget to meet. Although there would be a parent advocate at the meeting, she was provided by the school district, and I questioned whether she would, in fact, be an impartial observer.

At the meeting, as each educator summarized Miles's test results, it became apparent that Miles had not only caught up with his peers but that he was eight months ahead of age level for language, vocabulary, problem solving, social, and self-help skills. The CPSE chairman looked at me kindly.

"I'm sorry, he just doesn't qualify. He's doing better than fine. He's doing great."

"But—but . . ."

As his words sank in, my tears began to fall. I knew what he was saying to be true, and I began to realize that I could stop being so cautious and finally allow myself to believe it.

"I'm really sorry, I know you think he needs these services . . ." he began.

"It's not that," I said, trying to smile. "I'm crying because I'm starting to believe that it's over. This worry has become so much a part of my life, and now you're telling me that I have to learn to let it go."

The others in the room nodded their understanding. They had never seen a child with autism lose services before, and it was an important moment for all of us.

So there it was. I could not objectively decide if Miles, at three, had recovered from autism, but regardless, he did not qualify for services by a long shot. This meant that at the very least he had "achieved normal functioning," the very thing that I had hoped for after reading *Let Me Hear Your Voice.*

My attention turned back to the diet, and to the biological causes of my son's problem. Besides Jean Curtin, there were two other local moms from my group who were doing the same kind of research that I was: Kathy Terrillion and Jeannie McAllister. I could only assume that there were hundreds of others across the country. Our support group later grew to include over forty local families and became a chapter of a national Parents' Support Group for Children with Allergies. We met monthly to share information and lend support. It was such a relief to new members to know that they were not alone.

Soon, Kathy and Jeannie began to see a doctor in Buffalo, New York, who administered EPD injections to their children. EPD stands for enzyme potentiated desensitization. It is a series of a type of allergy shot intended to relieve food and environmental sensitivities. If all goes well, patients are reported to eventually be able to tolerate a wider variety of foods.

EPD sounded too good to be true. Wouldn't it be wonderful if Miles could eat soy, or even corn? There would be so many foods I could give him! As it turned out, EPD was effective for some of my friends' children, but I could not even consider starting the treatment at that time. For one thing, the doctor in Buffalo requested a complete overhaul of the household—ripping up carpets, installing special air filters, removing all new plastics and chemicals and cleaning products.

There I was again, resisting something new because it seemed like too much work. But my finances, for certain, could not withstand another expense.

As word spread about Miles, I began to be faced with a dilemma. My phone began to ring all the time, with parents calling from across the country for answers and advice. Most of them were wonderful to talk to, and had already begun to make some progress on their own. At first I enjoyed the opportunity to lend support. Soon it became a problem for me. Pre-educated parents were easy to help, but there were many who required an hour just to understand the basics of the intervention. I simply did not have the time.

But how could I say no? Each mother would call, describe her child, and ask some questions. It was always a challenge for me to make her understand what she might want to try. Several days later I would receive another call. Sometimes with tears in her voice, she would tell me of the differences in her child and express such profound relief that I had given her some hope. After a while I had heard so much feedback that I really was in an excellent position to give advice. Sometimes the stories were so much the same that the children seemed to merge into one:

Johnny eats only milk and/or wheat. He goes through a very cranky withdrawal when put on the diet. He improves. Other allergens begin to appear. He gets worse. Other foods are removed. He gets better. He begins nystatin. He has a die-off reaction and

gets worse, then improves dramatically. He gets contaminated with
wheat and gets worse. The diet becomes stricter and he further
improves. He begins to accept new foods.

I spent several hours with my notes, and the notes of Kathy and
Jeannie, and put together a huge information packet. I decided that
if a parent wanted to reimburse me for the photocopying, they could
read our notes for themselves before calling with questions. I was ada-
mant about not making a profit on the document, but soon learned
to regret that decision.

At first I mailed out about one packet a week. Soon it was two,
then three. Before I knew it, I had to get a post office box and give out
its number to the strangers who wanted to send me a check. I spent
hours each month getting copies made and mailed out.

At this time, I was running two retail businesses, a household, a
support group, and a very complicated family diet. My income was
minimal due to taking so much time off, my finances were a mess
from neglect, and we had overspent on Internet fees, specialty foods,
books, newsletters, phone calls, airfare to conferences, and increased
child care. In the one year since Miles's diagnosis, we had gone $30,000
deeper into debt. After that, because of the interest accruing on it, the
number went up to $40,000, then $50,000.

Those numbers made me feel dizzy, and a little sick. Looking at my
son, there was no question that what we had done had been worthwhile, even if it did eventually lead to bankruptcy. One parent had
told me that each autistic child costs his school district about a million
dollars over the duration of his education. What we had saved them
would now take us years to pay back, but I was not sorry. I had seen
others struggle with crises of their own, and I knew that life does not
always proceed the way we expect it to. I promised myself that if my
life ever returned to normal I would not complain about anything less
important than the welfare of my children.

Alan and I felt awful when we considered filing for bankruptcy, but in a way the idea made me feel calm, and almost relieved. People had done so for much less noble reasons, and if we did go bankrupt, we could start with a clean slate. Once it was over, I could finally stop worrying, and we could begin our lives again.

One of the worst problems was that my stores were not doing well. Without my supervision, payroll had gone up and profits were way down. Being there depressed me, too. There always seemed to be some eczema-covered, hyperactive child in the store drinking Kool-Aid from a bottle, or a two-year-old with no language and autistic behaviors, whose mother probably did not want to hear what I wanted to tell her. I needed a new job, but what I really cared about was something for which I did not want to accept payment.

I had to do something about the phone. It rang constantly, and I tended to drop whatever I was doing to answer it. Alan took me aside one evening and pointed this out. "You know, your family should still take priority over the rest of the world."

He was right. How many times had I stopped playing with Laura to answer the phone—and then stayed on for an hour?

I sat down the next morning and typed up a document that turned out to be a lifesaver: "Frequently Asked Questions About Dietary Intervention for the Treatment of Autism" (see Part Two, Chapter 9). Drawing on my experience with the many questions I had answered, I tried to cover the basics in a way that made it easy for even a beginner to follow. From then on, whenever a new parent called me, I was able to mail, fax, or e-mail the answers to most of their questions in just a few minutes.

Life started to get easier, then disaster struck. My sister-in-law was taken ill, and caring for her three children was becoming increasingly difficult for her. My brother's stepdaughter, Annabel, was having trouble with school and with her life at home. She was an aggressive eight-year-old who had not been diagnosed but who certainly had ADHD. Her parents asked if we could take her for a while.

I had no business taking on another project, but in my arrogance I was beginning to believe I could stop a snowstorm. I had been able to fight off my son's autism, hadn't I? Annabel's problem was probably related in some way to food allergy. Despite Alan's protests, Annabel came to stay with us in mid-February 1997.

During her first week I began to suspect that I had made a very serious mistake. This was the most hyperactive child I had ever met. She could not follow both parts of a two-part instruction. Not only couldn't she read, but she barely knew her alphabet. She talked, shrieked, and sang incessantly, and she drove all of us crazy. Annabel could not sit at the table without jumping up, could not get dressed without a dozen distractions, could not shut her mouth for more than ten seconds, and ate small amounts all day long.

Nystatin and probiotics (acidophilus and bifidus) seemed to help, and so did a diet low in sugar, but this was difficult to maintain. Annabel craved sugar and sneaked candy whenever she could, wherever she found it. Removing gluten and casein during her school break was easy enough, since my kids were doing it along with her, but it didn't seem to make a difference. I had only ten days before she went back to school, so perhaps I didn't give it enough of a chance, but my gut feeling was that it was not the answer. An allergy elimination diet also proved ineffective, although corn really seemed to worsen her hyperactivity, and avoiding it helped a little bit.

Susan Hyman stopped by for a visit. After watching Miles and chatting with him for a few minutes, her indignation that we had lost services from the school district dissolved. She agreed that Miles no longer seemed to meet many of the criteria for autism. She suggested that we schedule a time for her to formally perform two state-of-the-art tests to rate the disability: the ADI (Autism Diagnostic Interview) and the ADOS (Autism Diagnostic Observation Schedule).

I asked her for help with Annabel. Alan and I could not bear the thought of one more day with the child in our house, but we could not send her home until things stabilized there. I knew many children, many siblings of autistic children, with ADHD, who were able to function well after EPD or antifungal treatment, or a special diet. Many of them went off massive doses of Ritalin and never needed to go back.

But we had tried some of those things, and now it was time for me to consider Ritalin, or "vitamin R," as Alan jokingly called it, as an alternative for Annabel. Based on the results of the Conners Teacher Rating Scale (a simple evaluation that rates the severity of attention deficit) administered at school, Dr. Hyman agreed that Annabel far surpassed the minimum criteria for ADHD and was indeed a candidate for Ritalin.

In the circles of alternative medicine, where I now traveled, I knew that my conclusion was controversial and unpopular. Ritalin has many known and unknown side effects, and I did see it as an emergency measure, but for this particular child, Ritalin was nothing short of a miracle. Within three days we saw a spectacular difference in Annabel. When summer came, the child we sent home had a long way to go emotionally, but she was calmer, more introspective, and had learned that she could form real friendships with her peers.

My newest conclusion was that every child was different and that arrogance was the recipe for error. I had the nagging feeling that I could have done more to uncover the biological cause of Annabel's problem, but I simply had not had the time.

Still, was ADHD on the same spectrum as autism? Many people thought so, and my gut feeling was that many cases probably are a different form of the same disease, but possibly not in Annabel's case. At times she was totally oblivious to the effect of her behavior on others, but at other times she was painfully aware of our discomfort, her teachers' disapproval, and her classmates' disgust at behavior she simply could not control. I once heard that the immune system and the nervous system were closely linked; I felt certain that an immune insult was at the heart of both disorders.

Back to the question of what caused autism. I mulled it over for hours and hours and always came to the same conclusion: children were coming to the behaviors by different means, and this had to be why they required different treatments. So, what did they all have in common?

Then Alan came home from work one day with a strange expression on his face. "I think we've found something," he said, "something really, really weird."

CHAPTER SEVEN

Breakthroughs

Alan was a senior research scientist; he reported directly to the management level. As his work on an assay for urinary peptides progressed, he kept them informed on the outlook of his side project, as well as on the other work he was doing. Collecting urine samples from local autistic children, he and his assistant, Michelle, were intrigued to find peaks in the urine that did not appear in the urine of siblings or normal controls.

It seemed that Kalle Reichelt and Paul Shattock were correct—there did seem to be opiate-containing peptides in these children's urine that were breakdown products of gluten and casein, as well as a third peak that seemed to go down after a long time on the diet. But Alan's equipment was much more sophisticated than theirs. Using the company's state-of-the-art triple quadrupole electrospray mass spectrometer, he could identify each one of the peaks that had appeared using the less accurate high-performance liquid chromatography (HPLC) method. Whatever that mysterious substance was, he was sure to discover it.

But he was not prepared for the results. The urine samples he had taken contained something so unexpected, so harmful, that its presence in a human child seemed impossible. It appeared to be a known substance with strong neurological effects that had previously only been seen in the poison dart frog.

Alan was stunned. Dermorphin? Where the heck could that be coming from? It was a substance known to be so potent that the tiniest trace could have a powerful psychoactive effect. South American tribal shamans would hold one of these frogs over a fire to induce a stress response, then rub the animal's sweat secretions into an open cut. Then they would go into a hallucinogenic state that lasted for several hours.

If the smallest trace of dermorphin could induce such a state, why on earth were autistic children excreting it in large quantities?

Alan and his partner, John, double-checked the molecular weight of the substance to be certain. Once again, it checked out. It was astonishing but true—for some inexplicable reason, dermorphin could be bombarding the brains of human children.

I had heard of the poison dart frog, in a vague sort of way, but did not know much about it until Alan explained its history. "Holy cow," I said. "That sounds a lot more powerful than the casomorphin."

"That's not all," he continued. "After their hallucinogenic experience, the shamans are known to have terrible, profuse diarrhea."

"Wow. So that might be what's causing the autism, not the opioids from milk and wheat."

"Or a combination of the two. Or the production of the opioids could stimulate production of the dermorphin, which may disappear after some time on the diet. Or the same enzyme may be responsible for breaking down both, and this enzyme is not being utilized."

Further testing showed that this substance was present in many samples from autistic children, along with the gluten and casein peptides. In autistic children on the diet, it often appeared alone.

It was never present in normal controls, nor was it in our daughter, Laura's, urine. It was not present in Miles's urine, nor in that of one or two others who seemed to be on the road to recovery. In children who had responded well to the diet, it often appeared in small quantity. But in Larisa, who had been on a strict gluten- and casein-free diet for over a year, it appeared in great abundance.

Alan explained further. All of the endogenous (created from within) substances found so far in the human body contain an L-amino acid. Dermorphin contains a D-amino acid, which would suggest that it is not of human origin.

"If it's not human in origin, then what inside the body is producing it? Could it be a fungus or bacteria?"

"Well yes, that is a possibility. In the South American rain forest, dermorphin exists on the backs of this species of frog. When they are bred in captivity, they do not produce the substance. It doesn't appear to be part of the frog genome."

"What can we do to stop its production? How do you kill it? Can I tell Bill Shaw?"

"Slow down," Alan said. "This is diagnostics. Treatment comes later. Much as I would like to, we really can't talk about this or release the name of the substance until this has been published in a respected journal, or we submit the patent application."

"But—"

"But nothing. This is real science, real medicine. We need to test more patients, get them classified with a really reliable, standardized diagnostic technique, and conduct a clinical trial. If the research goes into the public domain, or becomes the property of the autism community now, before further research is done, my company will have to drop the project. Nothing is more important to the future of autism research than the necessity of secrecy at this time."

More waiting. The answers still seemed so far away.

"So, what should I tell people?"

"I'm not a doctor, so I can't make medical recommendations. You can tell parents that we've found evidence to support the importance of strict adherence to the diet, at least in many of the children. A course of antifungal treatment is not unreasonable. You can tell them that it may take time for the gluten and casein peaks to drop, and for other harmful substances to drop after the foods are removed. The ones who gave us samples can call Michelle to find out whether their kids may benefit from the diet. That is all they need to know to help their children. They don't need to know anything else right now."

"Alan, what do you think produced dermorphin in Larisa? She was on the diet for ages."

"That's a good question. My guess is yeast or anaerobic bacteria. Possibly not candida."

"Is there something I can suggest to Lori for her?"

"Well, she might as well continue the diet. Maybe it's just taking a longer time for Larisa's body to stop production. Lori could talk to her physician about a stronger antibacterial—perhaps something really powerful like vancomycin. But don't get too excited yet. The production of dermorphin may be very difficult to control. And for all we know, it could just be a marker for chronic diarrhea."

"Oh, come on, you're kidding, right?"

Alan smiled mysteriously and left me pondering this new information.

Well, that was it, then. Either the opiate peptides, anaerobic bacteria, or both, or neither, were triggering the production of dermorphin and its partner, a substance called deltorphin. For my child, done early enough, the diet (along with the nystatin, perhaps) had stopped production completely. For some children, long after implementation of the diet, the dermorphin and the autistic behaviors remained.

I went out to dinner with Terry Hines, the college professor who had given me my first real understanding of science and of neurobiology. He and I had become friends and had stayed in touch over the years.

Far from being skeptical, he listened with fascination as I told him about the urinary peptides and fungal metabolites in the bodies of children with autism. Perhaps it was because he trusted me to be skeptical myself, taught by him to carefully evaluate data for possible flaws.

"So," I concluded, "the only thing I really can't believe is that a fungus can produce a hallucinogen so potent that it could completely change a child's perception of the world." Terry thought about this for a fleeting moment, then gave me a wry grin. "Name the two most well known hallucinogens," he said.

"Um, well, LSD, and psilocybin."

"Source of LSD?"

"Uhhh, ergot, which is a *mold* that grows on rye, and psilocybin is from mushrooms that are . . . oh my God! A *fungus!*"

"Mmm-hmm."

"Terry, you're a genius. Why didn't I think of that?"

Of course. I should have seen it back when Shaw first spoke about yeast at that conference the year before. There were at least two precedents for the existence of a potent hallucinogen produced by molds.

So, this could be the source of the substance that Alan had identified. Now all we needed to know was how to get rid of it, and many cases of autism would be . . . no, wait, remember what I've already learned. It's never that simple.

Of course, this had to be a major piece of the puzzle. But the food allergies and the diarrhea were still elements for which I could think of several possibilities. How did the foods and the dermorphin get into the bloodstream? A leaky gut made sense, since something must have compromised the integrity of the intestinal wall, but what? Yeast? A virus?

Then, in a sample taken a few months later, the dermorphin peak finally disappeared from Larisa's urine. Miles was the first autistic child that Alan had tested to lose the peak and she was the second, and yet her autism remained. True, she seemed much better, and she no longer avoided contact with other children, but she still did not really use language to communicate. Was this because her brain had developed abnormally for five years? She had never had a "period of normal development."

Or was it because she had a different disorder than the others? The only thing that Larisa and Miles had in common was that their parents had strictly adhered to the diet for over three years. Did it take such strict adherence to make the dermorphin go away?

SPECIAL DIETS FOR SPECIAL KIDS

The very first time I spoke with Mary Cropley, I knew we would be friends. She called me after another parent gave her my number, and in a pleasant English accent she asked me about dietary intervention. I began to explain about the diet and asked if she had ever heard of gluten.

"Have I?" she asked. "Yes, I certainly have. I was diagnosed with celiac disease last year."

"Wow, that's great!" I blurted out, then realized how I sounded. "I mean, it's not great that you have celiac, but it's great that you will have an easy time understanding about the diet."

We arranged for Mary to stop by to watch Jill Pavone, our special-ed teacher, work with Miles before his services ran out. Although Mary's daughter, Annie, was over three, she had just been diagnosed; Mary and her husband, Dan, were still setting up a therapy program.

I answered the doorbell to find a beautiful, petite woman slightly older than myself, with blue eyes and brown hair pulled back in a bun, holding Annie by the arm with one hand and supporting David, her two-month-old infant son, in the other. She smiled, but worry lines creased her forehead.

Annie did not look around our living room, or head directly for the toys in the play area. She whined and pulled on Mary's arm, looking around just enough to perceive that the room was unfamiliar but not focusing on any one thing. Many autistic children had visited in the past year, and I had seen enough of them to recognize many of its manifestations. Annie was very fearful, and screamed when Mary moved even a foot away from her.

"Go!" she said, pulling her mother toward the door.

"Is Annie talking?" I asked, surprised.

"She was, which is why it took so long to diagnose her, but now I wouldn't say she's using language meaningfully—perhaps only a word or two."

Annie screamed when Mary put down the baby, screamed when she picked up the baby, and screamed when we took her upstairs.

"She's having a lot of trouble with transitions," Mary explained. "We want to start her in a special preschool, but I'm very much afraid that she won't be able to handle it. She has terrible separation anxiety when she's away from me."

Jill was working on a puzzle with Miles, who looked up, smiled, and said hello when we entered the room. Mary said that Annie liked puzzles, so Jill tried to work on a simple peg puzzle with her for a few moments, but Annie shrieked so pitifully at Jill's intrusion that I suggested we bring the puzzle with us and take her out of the room.

"I'm impressed with Miles," Mary said wistfully, settling on the couch downstairs and cradling David to nurse him. "You wouldn't know he had ever had a problem. You attribute it to diet?"

"Well, the therapy was very important, but we don't think it would have been successful without the diet. I highly recommend it for Annie, especially considering your celiac disease."

"I already know how to do a gluten-free diet, so I suppose I have no excuse. It just seems such a shame to take away her favorite foods."

"I know. And I'm going to give you some more advice that you won't like. I don't think you should let David have any gluten or dairy until he's much older, if ever, and you might want to consider postponing his vaccinations."

Mary sighed, but she nodded.

Mary became a very good friend that year. While she was from England, her husband, Dan, had grown up near Alan in Los Angeles. They had once lived near me in New York City, and we found that the four of us had a lot in common.

In addition, Annie responded beautifully to the diet. Within a few weeks she was less fearful, and instead of continuing to lose language, she began the process of regaining it. She loved school and began to form a strong attachment to her father. At Miles's birthday party a year later, she excitedly thrust a present into his hands, shouting "Hello, Miles! It's your birthday party!" She waited in line to whack at the piñata, asked politely for a second helping of gluten-free birthday cake, and grinned into the video camera and said "Happy birthday, Miles!" at my bidding.

Next to Miles and Bobby Ross, I had never seen a child with autism do so well. Again, I had to assume it was because of the length of the disease process before intervention. Annie was over two when her development slipped, and she had had a great deal of normal development under her belt before the problems arose. She also seemed to have been less severely affected than many, although in a few more months without treatment that might not have been true.

When Dan accepted a job in California, I was heartbroken. Mary was one of the few friends who understood what I had been through, and she was genuinely happy to see Miles's progress. She was the mother of another child spared by the Pied Piper.

Just before they moved, we took the children to the local zoo. Annie and Miles, who had a great affinity for each other, rode in the backseat.

"Annie, can we get married?" Miles asked matter-of-factly.

"Um, yes," she said quietly. I glanced into the rearview mirror and saw that they were holding hands and she was smiling.

"It would be good because we both can't eat gluten," Miles added.

"Okay."

I laughed, and told Miles he could write to Annie after she moved away, and that maybe they could marry once they were grown-ups. They both agreed that it was a good idea.

In September 1997, Lisa Lewis and I were invited to the third DAN! Conference in San Diego, to give a workshop on dietary intervention. Lisa and I had never met in person. Prior to the conference I had suggested that we collaborate on a support network for parents using the diet, the Autism Network for Dietary Intervention (ANDI). When we did come face-to-face, it seemed as though I already knew her well— she was like family. We shared a love of animals, cooking, and books, and we both soared to great heights over a simple thing like the discovery of a new gluten-free cookie recipe.

On the airplane to California, we exchanged information and I shared as much as I could about Alan's work, which was very little. I couldn't tell her about dermorphin yet, since Alan had made me promise not to. It was hard, but I trusted his judgment.

I was looking forward to meeting Kalle Reichelt, and to seeing Bernie Rimland and Bill Shaw again. Bill was working on a book called *Biological Treatments for Autism and PDD,* and Lisa and I had each contributed a chapter. I was pleased to participate in the conference, but I did not think I'd learn anything new. Then, on the second day of the talks, a good-looking Englishman stepped up to the podium and shook up my world once again.

A GASTROINTESTINAL DISORDER

I was embarrassed to admit it to myself, but if Dr. Andrew Wakefield had been talking about furnace repair, I probably would have paid attention. He spoke beautifully, with a confident, polished style of lecturing, and from the start it was clear that he believed what he was saying was very important. I was not the only one in the auditorium who noticed—there was absolute silence as we hung on his every word. Then, as his words got through to me, I began to listen even more eagerly.

Wakefield was a gastroenterologist. He had had several autistic children referred to him for chronic diarrhea and gastrointestinal disorders, and upon examination had found marked abnormalities.

Ileocolonoscopies revealed colonic and rectal mucosal abnormalities in eight of the twelve children, such as "granularity, loss of vascular pattern, patchy erythema, lymphoid nodular hyperplasia, and in two cases, aphthoid ulceration." This did not mean much to me, but I assumed it was not normal. Four of the cases showed an early endoscopic feature of Crohn's disease. Ten of the children were identified as having lymphoid nodular hyperplasia of the terminal ileum: somewhat common findings, but abnormal when compared with the images of the terminal ileum from seven normal controls. Tissue samples taken during the procedures were also abnormal when biopsied.

The children he described sounded just like Miles; they had chronic diarrhea and late-onset autism. Their parents sounded like me—discouraged and frustrated when physicians neglected the GI abnormalities because the child had autism, "that mysterious disease." Wakefield pointed out that a typical child with long-term diarrhea would have unquestionably been a candidate for a colonoscopy.

In addition, he reported that many of the parents of the children he saw indicated that they felt that the onset of the diarrhea and the autistic features had coincided with their child's MMR vaccine. He indicated that he needed more data to publish his findings, and then, as electricity virtually crackled in the air, he announced that his early results showed something that might actually substantiate their claim.

"We believe we have actually found measles antigen at the sites of disease in the bowel. Based on viral DNA comparisons, we believe its origin is the MMR vaccine, and that autism may be a gastrointestinal disease."

I thought hard, trying to remember. How old was Miles when he got his MMR? Fifteen months old? Wasn't that when his diarrhea started and his language disappeared?

Sharp images flew through my mind: At fourteen months old, Miles smiling and talking in Florida with my mom and playing drums at Sea World. Fifteen months old, eleven days after the MMR, in the hospital with his first round of febrile seizures. Three weeks later in California, my turning off the video camera after ten minutes of watching him pace back and forth across the same patch of gravel in the backyard. The pale little face in which a stony, unblinking stare had permanently replaced the sunny smile. Two months later, on the night of his DPT, another episode of seizures and my realization that he had lost eye contact.

Lisa was sitting next to me and I tried to say something to her, but when I opened my mouth, only a squeak came out. I looked at my hands—they were trembling. Oh God, what if this was true? Wakefield was presenting preliminary data, but something clicked in my brain. I experienced a moment of clarity in which every piece of the puzzle that was Miles's disorder slipped into place.

Before my eyes flashed every clue that I had ignored. Miles had probably had a milk allergy very early on, ear infections, parents with allergies and autoimmune diseases, long-term antibiotic use, and other reasons why someone should have questioned giving him so many antigens at such a young age. At four months old, having already had an adverse reaction to his last vaccination, he had been given a shot for diphtheria, tetanus, pertussis, haemophilus influenzae B, oral polio, and hepatitis B.

"Isn't that a lot to give a little baby all at once?" I had asked the doctor. "He's not going to be exposed to any of this stuff for a while."

"Oh no, it's standard procedure. We get them young so there's no chance that they'll slip through the cracks later on."

My child. Did I hold his little hand while the smiling nurse with the needle destroyed his gut and his immature immune system?

I thought of all of those wacky parents out there with bumper stickers that said say no to mandatory vaccinations. Terry Hines had taught me to laugh at such things, and I had dismissed it as alarmist propaganda. What if . . .

Whoa, Karyn, stop it. This was preliminary data and speculation. Just because it answered a lot of questions did not mean that it was true. But if it is true . . . suddenly, I realized the implications of what Wakefield was saying. When he published, every parent of an autistic child would be demanding colonoscopies and denouncing vaccinations. The British National Health Service and the U.S. Centers for Disease Control would have to prove him wrong or face a huge onslaught of legal settlements for vaccine damage. Not to mention the loss of the public's trust. Right or wrong, Wakefield did not have a chance.

I moved through the rest of the conference numbly, wanting to go home and look up dates and medical records.

Lisa and I gave our workshop on dietary intervention in a classroom that did not have enough seats for all of the parents wanting to try the diet and looking for practical advice. It seemed that after hearing Reichelt, Shaw, and Wakefield, there was a lot of interest from the parents at the conference. We handed out flyers for ANDI, the Autism Network for Dietary Intervention. We had printed five hundred, and every one had been taken by the end of the last day.

On the following morning I went home eager to talk things over with Alan. He agreed that after Wakefield's paper was published he would fly to England and discuss collaboration with him. Until then, he advised, keep your mouth closed and wait. I am not particularly good at either of those activities, but I promised to try.

Wakefield's paper, published in the February 28, 1998, issue of *The Lancet,* described a study involving twelve children with later-onset (after one year of age) degeneration of language and social skills (nine had been diagnosed with autism). Ten had developed typically until the MMR vaccination, one began symptoms of autism after an actual case of measles, and one after the onset of chronic otitis media two months after the MMR. All had been referred to a pediatric gastroenterology unit for diarrhea and abdominal pain, some with known food intolerances.

Wakefield concluded that his results, combined with other studies reporting intestinal dysfunction in autistic patients, indicated a "unique disease process" that needed to be studied further. He suggested that the impaired intestinal function that he observed could be responsible for the increased permeability that would allow for Reichelt's "opioid excess" (leakage of opiate-containing gluten and casein peptides from the gut into the bloodstream) theory to take place.

In addition, most of the children had elevated levels of urinary methylmalonic acid, which indicated a functional vitamin B_{12} deficiency. (Serum B_{12} levels were normal, but serum B_{12} is not judged to be a good indicator of functional B_{12} status.) Vitamin B_{12} is essential for the development of the central nervous system, a process that continues for the first ten years of life. This might explain why some children responded well to vitamin B supplementation.

His paper did not include his findings about the measles antigen. I assumed he was waiting for more data before he could confirm that the MMR definitely triggered the onset of autism, a theory that would most certainly threaten his career. When Alan called him to set up a meeting, Wakefield indicated that such a paper was forthcoming. But the mention of a possible MMR connection in *The Lancet,* without sufficient data to back it up, had been a mistake.

Wakefield received a tidal wave of criticism from the medical community. Letters poured in to *The Lancet* from all over the world, out-raged letters condemning the implication that vaccinations should be challenged. The national health departments of Great Britain and the United States both issued damage control statements that vaccines were safe.

"This is so ridiculous!" I told Alan after reading some of the letters that had been published in various papers. "The question isn't 'Should we vaccinate?' but 'Should we be screening out children who are at risk?'"

Alan smiled indulgently, as if expecting me to stamp my foot like an angry child. "We will," he said calmly. "Science and medicine take time. This will run its course. The truth will eventually preside over older beliefs. Thirty years ago autism was believed to be caused by bad parenting."

"Well, I know I sound petulant, but I hate feeling like some kind of subversive for thinking that we should clean up our vaccines, and stop culturing them in monkeys that are CMV positive, and that we should administer them one at a time, and to older children." I plopped down on my bed.

Alan tossed *The Lancet* onto the nightstand and sat down, but I jumped up again.

"I'm not waiting thirty years, that is unsatisfactory. Don't think I'm arrogant, because one person can make a big difference in the world. Look at what Portia has accomplished. Look at how many people have read Lisa's web page. Do you think that forty families in *this* city would be doing the diet if I had sat back and let it run its course? Would Bobby have a chance at a normal life if I hadn't talked Lori Ross into trying the diet before he was two? There is too much at stake for the families of young children with autism. These kids won't be so easy to have around the house when they're thirty-five."

Alan pulled me back down and put his arms around me. "Your passion is one of the things I love about you," he said. "But you don't have to save the world. Our family is important, too, and I really want to get on with our lives."

"I know. But please understand. I cannot move on with *my* life until I have reached some kind of closure with autism. Too many parents are suffering badly because their doctors don't know how to help them understand the diet, and Lisa Lewis is practically the only other person out there who is willing to do something. I know so much about this now, and I simply cannot rest until I have shared that information, and done it to my satisfaction. I know Miles has recovered, but I haven't."

Alan nodded. He would do his part, and see his project through to the end, and he would wait for me to do mine. But he looked at me wistfully.

One afternoon at the supermarket, I noticed a woman I had recently met at a party and waved at her. As she pushed her cart over to me I remembered that she had told me her four-year-old son had just been diagnosed with PDD but she was not interested in trying the diet. I didn't see the boy but there was a baby in the front of the cart sucking on a bottle. I remembered suggesting that she discuss postponing the baby's vaccinations with his doctor. She had reassured me that she had a wonderful pediatrician who was well educated about children with disabilities, and he thought the shots were okay.

"Hi," she said. "I was just thinking about what you said when I was over by the soy milk."

"Sally, right? Is this little cutie your younger son?" I asked.

"Yes, he's fifteen months old." She leaned on her cart and smiled.

"So, have you considered trying the diet?" I asked.

"Sort of. We decided that the first thing to do is try to get them to eat healthier, so we've been trying to cut out the junk food."

"No, I mean the dairy-free diet."

"Well, we had my older son off milk for about two weeks, since he likes rice and soy milk. We could definitely see a difference in him. Some days he seemed almost normal. But when we ran out we switched back. Anyway, he loves his ice cream so much that I really don't plan on taking that away. There are so few foods he'll eat as it is."

I remembered that I had described the opiate excess theory to her very carefully, explaining that this might be the reason her son's food choices were so limited. He would eat only cheese, macaroni and cheese, ice cream, and certain types of bread. I didn't like proselytizing about the diet once I had explained it to someone. I was tired of trying to convince people who didn't listen. But I took a deep breath.

"If taking *milk* away made a difference, don't you think it would be worthwhile taking away *all dairy*?"

"I suppose. But when I discussed it with my mother-in-law, she got really annoyed and said that your theory sounded crazy."

"It does sound crazy," I said. "In fact, in two or three years, when it has been proven, it will *still* sound crazy, and when your doctor tells you to put him on the diet, you will have lost two or three years. Are you going to blame that on her? It is your responsibility to act on this information, not your mother-in-law's."

"Yes, well, I am considering it," she said, confidently. "It's just that he loves cheese so much."

"My nephew would probably love peanuts," I said, "but if he ate one it would kill him." She actually laughed at this. Just then, her baby threw his bottle on the floor and then reached for it. "Ba!" he said. He was really cute. Sally bent down to pick it up.

"Don't lose this," she said to him. Then to me, she said, "We have hardly any bottles left and I don't want to buy more."

"Yes, he's at an age to switch to a cup," I agreed.

"Oh, no, he loves his bottle," she said. "He drinks milk all day long."

I took another deep breath and tried to smile through my frustration. Maybe milk was fine for that baby. Maybe he would have no reaction to his shots. But maybe he would. Part of me wanted to take him away, switch him to soy milk, postpone his vaccinations, and protect him from ignorance and blind faith in his doctor, just in case. His mother wasn't a bad person, and in another situation I might have liked her. How could I make her understand how critical it is to take full responsibility for your children's welfare?

I had recently had a similar conversation on the phone with another mom who had admitted that her inaction might have something to do with the fact that she was still somewhat in denial about the diagnosis. I had been very polite then, and sympathetic.

Later, thinking about her, I had felt very sad. Was there anything I could have said that would have helped her to take action, for the sake of her son? Should I have been less pushy? More authoritative? More pushy? No one has ever accused me of not being pushy enough, I thought. But Lisa Lewis, who was confident and straightforward, might have handled it better. Then Sally said something that almost made me fall over.

"It's only PDD," she said. I stared at her. There was a long pause.

"I can't believe no one has told you this before," I said, "but PDD is a severe, lifelong disability. PDD is autism." I took a step backward, startled by my own nerve. "Your son has autism, and if there is anything you can do to try to help, this is the time to do it."

She blinked at me a few times. She didn't look angry. It was hard to say if what I had said had even gotten through.

"Well, I suppose I could take away all of the dairy," she said. "But I don't think I'll be able to take away wheat." If I had a dollar for every time I heard that, I'd be a rich woman. How odd to hear someone say that she would go only so far to help her children.

"I'll tell you the difference between you and me," I said finally. "When I discovered that taking away *some* milk made a slight difference, I immediately took away *all* milk. When I discovered that gluten might be implicated, I took that away as well. It wasn't easy, but it was easier than spending the rest of my life with an autistic child. If you are in denial about this, I suggest you get out of it quickly, for your son's sake. It was nice seeing you again."

I trembled as I pushed my cart away. Later, I called Lisa and felt her anger rise as I described the incident.

"I know exactly how you felt," she said. "I've met a hundred like her. I always tell them that when their child's welfare becomes more important than their own convenience, that is when they'll be ready to do something. It's a harsh thing to say, but it's the truth."

A few days later, Miles suddenly awoke at midnight, crying out incoherently. He was trembling, and I remembered the nights of his seizures and panicked. I rushed him to the emergency room, where he appeared to be just fine. The doctor assured me that the episode was probably just a night terror, or the result of waking from a deep sleep. While waiting for the discharge papers, I noticed a notebook in the exam room labeled "Vaccine Adverse Reactions." I picked it up and discovered that there was a fund for children with vaccine damage, the Vaccine Injury Compensation Program.

The next day I called my friend Terri Kerr, the advocate of vaccine policy reform who swore that both of her sons' autism had begun with the MMR. She told me that if I decided to pursue it, I would need a lot of documentation to support my claim. She also told me that there was a three-year statute of limitations—this was March of 1998, and Miles's shot had been in the beginning of April of 1995. I had two weeks to file.

I called my lawyer and we talked it over. I had quite a bit of evidence that Miles's illness had coincided with the vaccine—I had videotapes, photographs, and two visits to the emergency room. But the

Vaccine Injury Compensation Program had plenty to lose if I won my case—there was a lot at stake. Did I really have a chance?

I felt so tired and worn out—I felt like I'd already given autism everything I had. But there were other children besides Miles out there whose parents were just as shaken, and they had not recovered. Was Miles's case strong enough to set a precedent?

My kid was better, sure; he was no longer autistic. But he had suffered terribly. All of that screaming, all of the pain he had been in. Four months of abnormal development that might affect his personality forever. A lifetime of eating a strict, sometimes costly, severely limited diet. And we were teetering on the verge of bankruptcy.

Damn. We had gone this far—we would have to go a little further.

Frantically, I began making phone calls, getting medical records from every doctor Miles had ever seen. On the night of April 4, 1998, my lawyer drove at top speed to the downtown post office while I sat in the passenger seat, sweating, numbering the pages in the binders we had filled. How the case would end, I couldn't even imagine. All I knew was that we had taken the first step.

Take that, vile beast, another blow from my sword.

At least I was no longer frightened by change.

COLONOSCOPY AND SECRETIN

Meanwhile, there was a new source of hope for treatment. Kelly Dorfman, the nutritionist who now specialized in the dietary needs of children with autism, had told me about an interesting development.

Secretin is an enzyme that, when infused into the bloodstream, causes the pancreas to release a flow of pancreatic enzymes, which can be collected and tested for insufficiency and function. When an autistic child in New Hampshire with chronic diarrhea was given a secretin infusion to test for pancreatic enzymes, his mother reported that he experienced a remarkable improvement both in his bowel movements and in his behavior.

After several weeks the benefits leveled off, and the mother, Victoria Beck, requested that the procedure be repeated. However, there was a hitch. Even though it was generally thought to be safe, secretin infusion was approved as a diagnostic procedure, not as a treatment.

This precaution is not as far-fetched as it sounds. The hormone used for this procedure is *porcine* secretin, derived from pigs. Just as diabetics can become intolerant to porcine insulin, it is possible that some people could develop an immune response to porcine secretin. Without data on repeated infusions, its safety was not guaranteed.

However, when news of Victoria's child's success spread, several other parents requested the infusion for their children. Many of those whose doctors agreed to it experienced similar results. Then, when the infusion was repeated, children who had responded sometimes showed further improvement, but many of their doctors were afraid of breaking FDA regulations by continuing the treatments. Dr. Rimland told me that studies were under way to explore the pathways that were being stimulated or possibly "unblocked" by the procedure, and that steps were being taken to make the treatment more readily available.

Victoria Beck, and other parents whose children had responded dramatically to a secretin infusion, were then on an episode of *Dateline,* the TV newsmagazine. When that happened, all hell broke loose. Parents all over the country who saw this and an opportunity to help their children bombarded their physicians with requests for an infusion. Susan Hyman told me that her office spent a week doing almost nothing but handling the influx of phone calls.

Alan commented only that the reported effects of secretin supported the theory that some forms of autism are gastrointestinal in nature, and that an enzyme deficiency may be present. When I asked for his recommendations about using secretin, he was very conservative. Once again, he simply said, "Sorry—I don't have enough data to form an opinion."

The following report was later released by Dr. Rimland at the Autism Research Institute:

Secretin Update from Dr. Rimland/ARI

Monday, January 11, 1999

The secretin story broke in early October. In quick succession, there appeared our secretin editorial in ARRI [*Autism Research Review International*] 12/3, Victoria Beck's superb presentation on October 3 at our DAN! Conference in Cherry Hill, N.J., and the *Good Morning America* and *Dateline* TV shows on October 6 and 7. Dozens of newspaper and magazine articles followed. The Ferring Company sold out of secretin by October 16. Parents, doctors, and university medical centers are scrambling to purchase new supplies as more secretin trickles into the pipeline. Efforts are under way to increase the supply.

The good news is that confirmatory evidence of the power of secretin keeps coming. A national newspaper told of Florida pediatrician Jeff Bradstreet's own four-year-old son, Matthew, shocking his parents by holding his first normal conversation with them the day after his first secretin infusion. And Virginia pediatrician Lawrence Leichtman told me of his "miracle case": a five-year-old who had previously said only two words amazed all in the office by saying, fifteen minutes after his infusion, "I am hungry. I want to eat." Most cases are much less dramatic, but the autism world is excited, and for good reason.

More good news, the Feds, including the FDA, are eager to help! Dr. Duane Alexander, director of the National Institute of Child Health and [Human] Development, and his assistant for autism affairs, Dr. Marie Bristol-Power, have been extremely helpful and supportive. I have been to two NICHD secretin meetings in Washington in the last thirty days, arranged by Dr. Bristol-Power. Following is the abstract of the presentation I gave at the December 14 meeting arranged by Dr. Bristol-Power to expedite the clinical trials the FDA requires.

The use of secretin appears to be the most promising treatment yet discovered for the treatment of autism. ARI has set itself the task of obtaining, as quickly as possible, at least tentative answers to the questions of greatest interest to parents and clinicians, and to researchers embarking on clinical trials.

Our Secretin Outcomes Survey (SOS) is a single-page questionnaire designed to elicit maximum useful information, with minimum effort, from the parents. The SOS has been distributed to parents of children undergoing secretin treatment through a variety of means:

Directly to parents, by mail or fax
Via physicians
In Victoria Beck's book
Via the Internet

To date, just over two hundred forms have been submitted to ARI, and more arrive daily. Many are incomplete or illegible (faxes don't like No. 3 pencils!), but most are useful and provide valuable data.

Here is what we have learned thus far. Obviously, these findings must be regarded as preliminary and tentative:

Q. Who is the best candidate for treatment with secretin? We don't know. We expected to find that certain categories of autistic persons would be more likely to show benefits than others; for example: low-functioning vs. high-functioning, those with diarrhea vs. those with normal bowel function, early-onset vs. late-onset, boys vs. girls, younger vs. older. So far, none of these anticipated predictors has proven valid, although there is a slight tendency for those with diarrhea to respond better behaviorally to secretin, but negligibly so. Judging from what we hear from physicians who have infused many cases (not from our SOS data) at least 75 percent (!) of their patients on the autistic spectrum show benefits from secretin, but we cannot yet identify a subgroup that does notably better or worse than the total group. Laboratory tests, such as blood secretin or blood ammonia levels, may prove predictive.

Q. What is the best dosage? We don't know. The Ferring Company suggests 1.0 to 2.0 Clinical Units of secretin per kg of body weight (for diagnosing digestive disorders—not treating autism), and that is what many have been given. However, our data include dosages ranging from 0.5 to 7.3 CU per kg. If we consider only those between 2.0 CU/kg and 5.2 CU/kg, disregarding the few cases at the extremes, there is no perceptible advantage to giving the larger amounts. There are slightly more negative reactions (e.g., hyperactivity) among those given the large doses. From present data, we would guess that a few years hence, when we know more, the optimal dose will be found to be between 2.0 and 3.5 CU/kg, on average, though some will need less and others more. (Some do well on 1.0 CU/kg.)

Q. What benefits are seen? Many, and they are benefits that are important in autism—eye contact, awareness, sociability, speech, and so forth. An unexpected benefit, better sleep, was a write-in, mentioned by many parents but not included among the choices we provided on the SOS form. Several children began sleeping the night through on the night of the infusion.

Q. What about adverse effects? About one-third of the children showed negative responses, mostly hyperactivity, and some aggressiveness, for a few days to a few weeks after the infusion.

In only a few cases were the problems severe. However, many autistic children have periods of disruptive behavior from time to time without secretin. In the absence of a matched control group of untreated autistic children, we have no way of knowing whether the problems actually were, in any or all cases, caused by secretin. There is speculation that behavior problems are more likely to be seen in the children on drugs, especially seizure drugs, but we have too little data to confirm or refute this, and other possibilities.

Q. What is the optimal schedule of administration? We don't know—too little data as of yet. Some say five to six weeks, but we don't really know. Our data do tell us, however, that the benefits, when they occur, can start quite quickly and seem to peak, in terms of percentage of children who respond, at about the end of the second week. Thus, we have been telling clinical researchers that the optimal delay between infusion and evaluative testing is about two weeks.

Other questions: While the dim outlines of the answers to some of our questions are beginning to emerge, we need much more data in order to come up with needed information. Among the outstanding questions:

Age: How well do adolescents and adults respond to secretin? It is too early to be sure, but it is beginning to appear that teenagers and adults improve as well as the children.

Repeat infusions: If the first and/or second infusions do not show significant benefit, is it worthwhile to try again?

Relapses: How long until relapse if secretin is discontinued, and do some improvements relapse faster than others? While, as mentioned above, five weeks is sometimes mentioned, we really don't have a good answer to these questions.

Adverse effects: What causes adverse effects? Do drugs, diets, infections, and other factors influence outcome? We don't know.

Parents and physicians are urged to help our data collection efforts. We will share what we learn.

If you would like to fill out the SOS questionnaire, go to: http://www.autism.com/ari/sos.html.

Alan went to England and met with Andrew Wakefield, and they agreed to collaborate. He looked at pictures of the swollen nodules in the terminal ilea of the children Wakefield had scoped, and discussed future research options. He phoned me from the hotel to fill me in. I was full of questions.

"You said that Wakefield thinks that in the kids he studies, diarrhea and constipation are occurring simultaneously, right?

"Well, that they are mostly constipated, and the diarrhea that we see is what leaks past the mass that is blocking up the intestine. This doesn't apply to all of the kids, but GI symptoms of some kind really do seem to be common. Remember, dermorphin might cause diarrhea, but codeine is constipating. So are many other opiates."

"Wow. This might explain why so many of the parents complain about constipation, not diarrhea. Do you think that what he's found is convincing?"

"Yes, definitely. But he needs more data. Real science means that *theory* doesn't become *fact* until it has been duplicated. Wakefield is going to have to proceed very carefully."

When he returned from England, Alan agreed to let Miles's new pediatric gastroenterologist, Dr. Medlow, do a colonoscopy. "Although," he warned, "Wakefield's patients were not on a gluten-free diet at the time of the colonoscopy. Miles's colon may have looked like that two and a half years ago, but it probably won't now."

Dr. Medlow agreed, but in light of the fact that Miles's diet was still just as limited as ever, and that his stools were still quite thin and loose, she felt that a colonoscopy was not a bad idea. She agreed to test his pancreatic enzymes with a secretin infusion during the procedure.

The first thing we did was an upper GI series. This involved Miles's drinking a barium mixture and undergoing a series of X-rays to make sure that the process of food reaching his stomach, and the juncture between the small and large intestines, was normal. I called the lab beforehand and discovered that the barium drink contained wheat, despite the fact that it is often used for people with celiac disease. They promised to order it in its pure form, so that I could bring a milkshake for Miles and add the barium when we arrived at the hospital.

Although this procedure took several hours, Miles was a good sport and had no trouble drinking the DariFree milkshake with the barium. I recalled that the regular sickly sweet and chalky form was almost undrinkable, and commented to the technician that this should be offered as a regular option for young children.

The colonoscopy was much more of an ordeal. Miles had to fast for a full day beforehand and cleanse his bowel with a bottle of magnesium citrate that evening. Again he surprised us by handling this very well. We explained that the doctor was going to try to fix his allergies so that he could eat more foods, and he settled for water instead of food. Since he was going to have diarrhea anyway, I tried offering him some punch, but he balked at the unfamiliar flavor. That evening I bribed him to drink the mag citrate with a bag of toy superheroes I had picked up at a garage sale and had saved for the occasion.

The following morning there was no sign of Miles's usually sparkling personality. He lay limply in my arms as I lifted him from the car and carried him through the hospital's ramp garage. He did not even have the strength to speak, but managed a smile when he saw Alan in the waiting room. Then I heard him whisper, "I have to throw up," and had enough time to prepare for a small amount of clear, liquid vomit. My heart ached for this little child, and what he had to endure, and for his bravery and innocence, and his trust.

I had prepared his inner arm with a numbing cream, and he did not flinch when the IV needle was inserted. Moments later, Miles was asleep.

The procedure went well. The pictures of Miles's colon looked normal and healthy. In the terminal ileum there were indeed a few nodules, neat round swellings with pink nipples in the centers. They were spaced like a row of suckers on the tentacle of a piece of calamari.

However, as such they were not an extremely abnormal finding. What they had looked like when Miles was first diagnosed, I wished I knew. The doctor took some tissue samples for culture, and told us that she would have the results in a few days.

Miles and Laura were eating lunch when I answered the kitchen phone.

"Most of the tests came back normal, but I was rather surprised at the amount of bacteria we found," said Dr. Medlow. "Usually, the small bowel is rather sterile, but we found massive colonies of anaerobic bacteria. *Pseudomonas aeruginosa, Escherichia coli,* and *Stenotrophomonas maltophilia,* to be specific."

"What about yeast?" I asked.

"Very little," Dr. Medlow replied.

"Maybe because we've had him on nystatin for three years?" I pondered. "What do we do about the bacteria?"

"Let's give him ten days of Flagyl, and see if he can eat a bit more variety. It's possible that there was some irritation from the bacteria that caused the problems."

"Okay. How about if I send Shaw a urine sample and see if it correlates with what you found, then repeat his test after the Flagyl? Maybe I'll even repeat it again after a month or so, to see if the bacteria comes back."

"That sounds like a good plan—please send me the results. Also, Miles has alactasia. That means he produces no lactase at all. Lactase is the enzyme that digests milk sugar."

"Could that be because he has been off dairy for three years?" I asked.

"Possibly. It's unclear whether he ever produced lactase at all. I don't know whether that is related to his other problems, however."

When I told Miles that there was some medicine that might help him to eat more foods, he put down his spoon and looked stoic.

"Well, even if it's really icky, I'll still take it."

I was pleased to see that Miles's urine test results from Dr. Shaw's Great Plains Laboratory *did* correlate with Dr. Medlow's findings: they reported very little yeast and a lot of bacteria. We gave Miles the Flagyl for ten days, fearing a die-off reaction, but there seemed to be little difference in his temperament. If anything, he was in fine form, and his stools looked unusually good—perhaps because of the secretin he had been given during the colonoscopy. Or perhaps because his bowels had been cleansed by the magnesium citrate. It was hard to say.

After treatment I collected a second urine sample to send Bill Shaw, and we decided to stop giving Miles the nystatin. The sample showed a dramatic reduction in bacteria, and two months and ten months later other samples showed no increase in either bacteria or yeast.

The outcome of the treatment? Our tentative introductions of new foods indicated that Miles's options had expanded slightly. His stools darkened and became firmer. We continued to be meticulous in our avoidance of gluten and dairy, but found that small amounts of egg, soy, and chocolate did not produce adverse reactions. Cautiously, we rotated these, in small amounts, into Miles's diet, again with no ill consequences.

I purchased a secondhand electric ice cream maker at a garage sale, and Miles enjoyed many different flavors of a frozen concoction made from the DariFree potato milk: mint chocolate chip, coconut-carob, vanilla-mango, and more. He was utterly delighted. I was amazed. A lifetime on a gluten-free diet would be easy compared with the limitations he had had for so long. Unfortunately, we found that corn was still a big problem and, as a result, were reluctant to try other foods.

So, was it the secretin or the Flagyl, or both, that improved Miles's reactive GI system? Perhaps it was the three years he had spent without gluten, perhaps letting his gut lining heal. It seemed that he could eat more foods, but we were afraid to push the limits to the point of a reaction. We did not rule out further treatment with gluten-free Asulfadine, a medication that helps to neutralize allergy basophils that line the gut wall, but that was still experimental for subjects like Miles, and in rare cases patients have had severe allergic reactions to the drug.

A month later the effect seemed to have worn off. Miles's stools were once again thin, light yellow, and loose.

Three months later, four other families that we knew had taken their children to Dr. Medlow. In some of the ones who had a colonoscopy, she found severe colitis and other abnormalities greater than Miles's. Dr. Medlow, once pleasantly skeptical, now agreed that there were preliminary data to support Wakefield's thesis: that there was some evidence of gastrointestinal abnormality in autism. She emphasized that a great deal of further testing would need to be done before she could draw any conclusions about the connection.

In October 1998 I attended the fourth DAN! Conference, in Cherry Hill, New Jersey, where Lisa and I were once again asked to give a parent workshop. Victoria Beck was there, speaking about secretin, and Dr. Wakefield was there, with an update on his research on autism and abnormal colonoscopy. He had more impressive data now, having scoped many more children, and identifying the presence of measles antigen in many more of the biopsy samples.

Alan had been asked to speak, too, presenting his data that confirmed the presence of gluten and casein neuropeptides, and breaking the news about dermorphin. He theorized that a deficiency in an enzyme called CD26, also known as DPP-IV, could result in such a pattern. DPP-IV is utilized for T-cell activation, which is a function of the immune system. I remembered from the 1996 DAN! Conference that one of the researchers had noticed abnormalities of T-cell activation in autistic children. Another of DPP-IV's known functions is to break down casomorphin, the opiate peptide derived from milk.

Most companies insist that proprietary information be kept confidential, to protect them from others who might steal their ideas. Luckily, it is part of Johnson & Johnson's credo that its employees should not withhold information that could immediately benefit the public: especially so in the case of children. So when Alan announced that his group at J&J had confirmed Reichelt's and Shattock's findings, and were planning to publish their results in 1999, the crowd burst into applause. I was sitting next to Paul Shattock during Alan's talk, and I hugged his arm.

"I've been waiting a long time to hear this," I whispered.

"Me, too," he replied. He handed me his handkerchief and I realized that I was crying.

CHAPTER EIGHT

Moving Forward

Dr. Kopelson had reported to me that many of his patients had achieved exciting results with an intravenous secretin infusion, while only a few did not improve. He couldn't guess at the percentage of the general autistic population that would respond, since his patients were self-selected. Although it seemed at first that the best candidates for secretin were those with a known GI dysfunction, he now believed that this did not necessarily turn out to be a predictor of good results.

Lisa Lewis's book came out, and it was a huge success. It was a tremendous relief to be able to answer parents who were looking for help with a single sentence: "Buy the book—it has everything you could possibly need to know about the diet." I was very proud to be working with her, and to have contributed to *Special Diets for Special Kids*.

William Shaw's book *Biological Treatments for Autism and PDD* sold seven thousand copies in just the first few months after it was released. The information was getting out, and I knew that a parent at the point of diagnosis had a better chance at discovering this treatment than I'd had.

Larisa's mother, Lori, told me that she had started her daughter on a homeopathic tea from the Ojibwa Native Americans and some other homeopathic remedies. Homeopathy was something I had not yet explored, and I decided to find out more about it.

According to *Merriam-Webster's Collegiate Dictionary* (11th ed.), homeopathy is "a system of medical practice that treats a disease esp. by the administration of minute doses of a remedy that would in healthy persons produce symptoms similar to those of the disease."

Miranda Castro, R.S. Hom., author of *The Complete Homeopathy Handbook,* 1990, defines it as "The Similimum or Law of Similars: This basic law of homeopathy is *similia similibus currentur*: 'let likes be cured with like.' Based on this premise, the first homeopathic principle states that any substance that can make you ill can also cure you—anything that is capable of producing symptoms of disease in a healthy person can cure those symptoms in a sick person. By 'symptom' the homeopath means those changes that are felt by the patient (subjective) or observed (objective), which may be associated with a particular disease, or state of dis-ease, and which are the outward expression of that state."

A further definition, by Stephen Cummings, M.D., and Dana Ullman, M.P.H., authors of *Everybody's Guide to Homeopathic Medicines,* originally published in 1991, stated: "Homeopathy is a 200-year-old medical system you can use at home to help treat family members with a wide spectrum of acute health problems. It offers a way to gently stimulate your inner healing resources through recognizing and reinforcing the adaptive reactions of the body's natural defenses. By choosing the correct, individually suited homeopathic medicine from the plant, mineral, animal, or chemical kingdom, you can successfully stimulate the body's own defenses . . . you can complement your family's efforts toward good health with these safe, natural medicines that provide an effective, inexpensive alternative to conventional medicine."

I had not explored homeopathy, because it really went against the grain of what I had been taught by Dr. Hines. But I had not ruled it out as possibly useful, and was interested to hear what Lori had to say.

Over the first three months, Lori and Steve had observed marked changes in Larisa's behavior, and her bowel movements had become much more normal in color and texture. Larisa was now able to eat a greater variety of foods without a reaction.

"Do you think it is doing something for the digestion?" I asked.

"I'm not sure, but Jean Curtin calls it a detoxifier. I think it's an immune system booster. You have to start with a really small amount or you can have a really toxic reaction. Some of the moms have improved on it as well."

I went to visit Lori the following week, thinking about the stony-faced little girl who had never really left my thoughts since the beginning of my ordeal. She was so different from Miles, so lost and locked away. Testing had shown her to have no antibodies to candida, her immune system seemed to be abnormal, and she had responded to dietary intervention, but her gains had been so slow. She was now five and a half, three months older than my son, and a world away.

Larisa's little face peeked out through the front window as I walked up the path to the door. That alone surprised me. But when Lori opened it, the little girl actually smiled at me.

"Say hi," Lori prompted.

"Hi!" Larisa looked at me as she spoke brightly.

"Hi, sweetie!" I replied, startled. Larisa had said hello before, but always while looking away, and in a low monotone. She then grabbed my hand and pulled me to the couch. I tried to remember if the child had ever touched me before. I recalled that she had always drawn away.

Then she picked up a toy horse and plopped down next to me, her thigh touching mine. "Hoss!" she said. "G'yup. Ba-bum, ba-bum, ba-bum." The horse pranced across our knees. A tear, which I tried to blink back, sprang to my eye.

"My God, Lori, is this from the tea?"

"I don't know. It has coincided with us giving it to her. Yesterday, I found her sitting on the potty. When I came in, she looked up and said, 'Pee-pee, poo-poo.' She was wearing a diaper, but she really seemed to understand. She's never done anything like that."

"And she can eat more foods?"

"Yes, almost everything. I've been reluctant to give her dairy and gluten, of course."

"Gosh, I wish I really knew what was going on. Could the tea be increasing T-cell function? Is it releasing a human form of secretin? Is it soothing the nervous system? Neutralizing IgG allergic reactions?"

"I wish I knew. I would have been reluctant to try the tea, but I've heard this from so many of the other moms in the group, too. Kathy and Jean and Elinor have also seen results with their kids. Some of the moms with fibromyalgia are taking it themselves. In fact, Kathy looks great—you should see her."

Larisa climbed into my lap and gave me a tight hug, then smacked her lips near my face. "Kisses," she said.

I blinked several times. "I guess this is the next step for me, then," I said weakly. "Blast off to the outer limits."

In 1999, while checking my e-mail, I read a notice on the CAN Parent Advisory Board listserv regarding a proposal from F. Edward Yazbak, M.D., FAAP.

Is There a Relationship Between the MMR Vaccine and Autistic Syndromes?

Dear Friends,

Two recent studies have shown that during this decade there has been an alarming increase in the incidence of autistic syndromes in the United States. Both studies have also suggested that this increase will accelerate in the coming years. Because the "outbreak" is so recent, we have postulated that:

Certain families seem to have a genetic predisposition to a fragile immune system. When a mother is repeatedly exposed to certain antigens or toxic environmental factors, she develops antibodies against them, which she transmits to her children. If the immature immune system of those children is attacked, early in life, by several simultaneous antigenic insults, violent complex immune reactions take place, which affect their whole body, and particularly their actively growing brain centers, leading to autism.

For the past few years, many parents of autistic children have reported a temporal relationship between the administration of the MMR vaccine to their children, and the onset of their symptoms.

To date, spokespersons for the CDC (Centers for Disease Control and Prevention), pro-vaccine groups, and vaccine manufacturers, have all adamantly denied any such link. The many studies which they quote in support of their argument, including one just published this week, have been, in return, rejected by the parents' groups, because of flaws in design, unsupported conclusions, short follow-ups, and the fact that some are funded by vaccine manufacturers.

It is therefore obvious that, because of this polarization, and the present, very peculiar set of circumstances, it has been impossible to prove or disprove that the MMR vaccine contributes, or has contributed, to the increase in autistic disorders.

Prospective studies cannot be done because of all the vaccine mandates. Retrospective-case controlled studies have to include huge numbers of patients, and require a lot of time, effort, and resources. Health and vaccine authorities have no interest in undertaking such extensive studies, which may lead to a causal relationship between MMR and autism—a relationship they deny.

We are a team of independent investigators trained in pediatrics and infectious diseases. We are not looking for, and we will not accept, any financial gain from this study, nor from any other work we do, in the fight against autism. We would like to investigate one unique aspect of the MMR controversy, never examined to date.

Some mothers who have been immunized as youngsters against

measles, mumps, and rubella, either with single vaccines or with the MMR, are found to have inadequate rubella (German measles) titers when they are tested before marriage, or during a pregnancy. I believe that the lack of protective antibodies is not due to a problem with the vaccine, but actually to a problem with the immune system of the woman herself, an abnormality that she could pass down to her children. In the past it was believed that this lack of protective antibodies was due to a problem with the vaccine itself. Therefore, an additional MMR booster is then administered, usually at an appropriate and recommended time. Even after that booster, however, some of these mothers still do not show immune titers of rubella antibodies, so another MMR is administered, and sometimes yet another. Similarly, many women starting college are required to receive an MMR booster, regardless of their immune status, and/or examination of their existing disease titers.

We think that it is possible that some of these mothers have produced sky-high titers of antibodies against measles, which they subsequently have transferred to their children. (Note that they could have already had adequate or high measles antibody titers, before the MMR booster or boosters.)

Distinguished investigators in the United States have demonstrated extremely high measles and/or rubella antibody titers in mothers of autistic children (and in the affected children themselves). If we can identify a large number of mothers who have received such MMR boosters, we can then look and see if they were more likely to have autistic children.

To participate in this study, you must have had measles or received, for any reason, an MMR vaccine as a booster after the age of sixteen, and be a mother of an autistic *or* nonautistic child.

I learned that Dr. Yazbak was a board-certified pediatrician who had been in practice since 1964. He had served as director of pediatrics at Woonsocket Hospital in Rhode Island, assistant clinical director (pediatric infectious diseases) of the Chapin Hospital in Providence, Rhode Island, and deputy director for pediatrics for the Child Development Study at Brown University.

His theory made some sense to me, especially in light of the fact that I had not retained a rubella titer and had received so many MMR vaccines. I was sure about having one when I was twelve and again at twenty-six when I was trying to get pregnant with Laura. Then of course, at twenty-eight, four hours after Miles was born. I also vaguely remembered having a measles shot when I was seven, and another MMR when I entered college. Yikes.

Dr. Yazbak had supervised four polio and other infectious diseases wards; worked closely with CDC field teams investigating a polio and a viral meningitis epidemic; coordinated the first statewide polio immunization program in the nation; participated in the training of pediatric residents in infectious diseases, carrying out all immunization mandates; and coordinated with his local Department of Health two citywide vaccination campaigns to control a measles and a meningococcal meningitis outbreak.

And now, after two of his grandchildren were diagnosed with autism, he was determined to find out if there could be a connection between autism and vaccinations. He had joined the Autism Autoimmunity Project, a public, nonprofit charity funding independent research into autoimmunity and autism.

The main reason autism is officially suspected of being an autoimmune disorder is due to the work of Vijendra K. Singh, Ph.D. He found that 60 percent of autistic children test positive to myelin basic protein (MBP), indicative of an autoimmune condition.[*] He has also

---

*V. K. Singh et al., *Brain, Behavior and Immunity* 7 (1993): 167–73; V. K. Singh, *Journal of Neuroimmunology* 66 (1996): 143–45; V. K. Singh, *Progress in Drug Research* 48 (1997): 129–46; V. K. Singh et al., *Clinical Immunology and Immunopathology* 89, no. 1 (1998): 105–8.

identified problems of interleukin-12 (IL-12) and interferon-gamma (IFN-g), two key proteins of the immune system that cause autoimmune diseases.

In June 1999, researchers led by Dr. Anne M. Comi of the Johns Hopkins Hospital in Baltimore reported that study subjects with a strong family history of immune disorder were twice as likely to have autism compared to subjects without such histories.* The researchers compared rates of various autoimmune disorders in the families of sixty-one autistic patients and forty-six healthy controls. They reported that families with two or more members suffering from autoimmune disease faced double the risk for autism compared with families without such histories. And the risk increased further when more family members were affected. "Those [subjects] with at least three family members with autoimmune disorders were 5.5 times more likely to have autism," according to the authors.

The investigators also point out that having a mother with some form of autoimmune disease raised individual risks for autism nearly ninefold. The autoimmune illnesses most often associated with raised risks for autism include type 1 (early-onset) diabetes, rheumatoid arthritis, hypothyroidism, and lupus.

I was not at all surprised by this. A lot of time was being spent searching for the "autism gene," when it seemed so obvious to me that a genetic predisposition toward immune system dysfunction was the groundwork for the ultimate condition of autism.

The recipe was simple: start with a child from a family like mine and add cow's milk, ear infections, long-term antibiotics, diphtheria (3x), tetanus (3x), pertussis (3x), haemophilus influenzae B, oral polio (2x), hepatitis B, measles, mumps, and rubella before the first eighteen months, then let simmer until all language and social skills have disappeared.

---

*Journal of Child Neurology 14 (1999): 388–94.

I printed up a copy of Dr. Yazbak's survey to fill out, spent a few minutes looking through my reference books, and wrote him a quick e-mail.

Dear Dr. Yazbak,

I am researching the dates of my MMRs—I'll fill out your survey in a week or so and get it back to you. I will also forward the survey to some other moms. I was last vaccinated with the MMR when my son was less than one day old, and he was breast-feeding. He later became autistic in the three weeks following his MMR at fifteen months.

I found the MMR vaccine under "Merck," in the *Physician's Desk Reference*. Here's what they say:

"It is not known whether measles or mumps vaccine virus is secreted in human milk. Recent studies have shown that lactating postpartum women immunized with live attenuated rubella vaccine may secrete the virus in breast milk and transmit it to breast-fed infants. . . . Caution should be exercised when MMR-II is administered to a nursing woman."

He replied:

Hi Karyn, I was well aware of the above. Were you informed of that "caution"? You should get a copy of this huge CDC manual for your library: *Epidemiology and Prevention of Vaccine-Preventable Diseases*. You can request it from the Public Health Foundation at 877-252-1200 or 800-41-TRAIN. The January 1999 issue, page 185, states: "Breastfeeding is not a contraindication to rubella vaccination and does not alter rubella vaccination recommendations." However, under "Rubella," they just talk about MMR as if the rubella vaccine does not even exist alone, so the risk of the measles-mumps portion of the vaccine during breastfeeding is not addressed. Earlier in the section, it says "Postpartum Women: It has been found convenient in many instances to vaccinate rubella-susceptible women in the immediate postpartum period."

I notice this says "convenient," not "safe."

I decided to get my measles antibody levels checked. It won't be much of a surprise if they are sky-high, I thought, glumly. What if this was the reason that the MMR triggered Miles's autism, whereas so many typical children do not react to the vaccine?

Later, when I spoke with Dr. Yazbak about his preliminary findings, he told me that he was quickly coming to the conclusion that any live, attenuated virus should not be given to women after their late teens, especially before, during, or after a pregnancy. He also informed me of new research about interferon gamma, a substance shown to be produced after MMR vaccination, which is known to lead to increased permeability of the intestinal tract and the blood-brain barrier. Interesting.

The precise connection among secretin, dermorphin, gluten, and casein are still not understood, and we need to have the answers to many questions. For the time being, the DAN! physicians' treatment recommendation is to carefully omit gluten and casein from the diet for a long period of time, perhaps in combination with taking an antifungal such as nystatin. Only after two to three years on the diet did the peak disappear in a few of Alan's subjects, with Miles, Larisa, and Annie included. My guess is that it was probably true of Bobby Ross as well, who did not have a second urine test but was in a regular preschool, looked wonderfully nonautistic, and would almost certainly succeed in a regular kindergarten by the time he turned five.

Despite the fact that Miles had had a reaction to his two-month DPT and was hospitalized with seizures after his fifteen-month MMR and eighteen-month DPT, and despite the fact that we had carefully put together medical, video, and photographic documentation of his autistic regression during the four weeks following his MMR, our vaccine claim was dismissed for "lack of evidence." I was shocked but I shouldn't have been surprised. If anything, I had hoped that the mere fact that his chronic gastrointestinal problems had been triggered by the MMR would at least warrant some compensation. In 2008, however, the federal government agreed to award damages to the family of Hannah Poling, a girl who developed autism after receiving the DTaP, Hib, MMR, varicella, and polio vaccines in one day. In her case it was determined that vaccines hadn't caused her autism, only triggered "autistic-like symptoms" due to a preexisting mitochondrial disorder. Whether other children whose parents report post-vaccination regressive autism also have preexisting mitochondrial disorders is unknown.

The future of our stakes in a class-action lawsuit (undertaken by families who also felt that the MMR was responsible for their children's autism) is yet to be determined. Miles had been a typical child, perhaps with allergies and a mild language delay, at the age of fifteen months. His social deterioration had occurred between that time and the day we took him off dairy at nineteen months old. Therefore, there was only a four-month period during which his body had battled the onset of autism.

Functionally, it set his development back to infancy. It took him almost two years of intensive training to relearn skills that he had lost and to catch up with his peers. But biologically, the disease process had still been reversible: an almost unheard-of phenomenon. This proved one thing to me that had to be shared with other families: that some cases of autism were treatable with dietary intervention, and the sooner, the better.

Miles had potty-trained himself at three and a half, with no prompting from us, and had never had an accident. He became very close to our two consecutive au pairs, Cheryl and Sue, and sometimes asked to call them on the phone after each had returned to England. He drew pictures for me to mail to them. He was deeply attached to his sister, and tried to do everything as well as she did. He picked out his clothes each morning, dressed himself, learned to pump on the swings and ride a two-wheeler, helped make his special cookies, and asked for a lullaby every night before he could go to sleep.

Dinosaurs were still an interest, but not a passion. Miles loved his "big-kid" bike, splashing in the kiddie pool with Laura, and playing Monopoly Junior. He had a "best friend" on our street and a "girl-friend" at school. He had a great sense of humor, "getting" riddles that used puns, loving tongue twisters and knock-knock jokes.

Susan Hyman had done the ADI when Miles turned four, and he had scored negative (that is, not abnormal). On the formal adminis-tration of the ADOS he scored normal in the social areas, with mildly abnormal eye contact and some borderline differences in pragmatic language. Susan knew him well and assured me that she did not be-lieve that the test reflected his actual verbal ability. She wrote:

Although I am quite confident in our initial diagnosis of an Au-tism Spectrum disorder in Miles at age two, his current presenta-tion would not lead a diagnostician to express any developmental concerns. The history obtained for the ADI-R did not reach cri-teria for a diagnosis of autism. Similarly, on the ADOS-G he did not reach cutoff scores for clinical concern. Both protocols were assessed for reliability with a rater who did not know the clini-cal history. Miles is currently functioning at an age-appropriate level and does not appear to have any developmental or behavioral problems.

Aside from the fact that he always had to be reminded to put away his toys and clothes, Miles was so sweet and good that it was almost unnerving. He had an uncanny perception about when to use his best manners, when to lie low during an argument, and when to use charm to get his way. Once, when I was in a terrible mood, banging dishes, yelling at the children and Alan about the mess in the house, Miles slipped off his kitchen stool and held up his little arms: "Mommy, I think you need a hug."

When Miles was four and a half, we visited my friend Mary Cropley and her husband, Dan, in San Diego, where they had moved. Little David was almost two, and he had become one of the most delightful children I had ever seen. He was extremely sociable, imitative, and affectionate. He was somewhat language-delayed, using only a few nouns, but he was so clearly nonautistic that it just didn't seem to matter. He sat on my lap giggling while we played a couple of bouncing games.

"I wonder if this is what Miles would have been like if it weren't for his vaccination," I speculated. "A little delayed, and probably genetically susceptible, but wonderful. Maybe this is what Alan was like as a baby, and that's why I find David so irresistible."

"Hmm." Mary smiled. "Oh, I forgot to tell you—remember how worried I was about getting David and Annie into school without their vaccines?"

"Yes, why?" I replied.

"In California it's barely a problem. All you have to do is check a box saying that you exempt them for personal reasons, and that's it. If there is an epidemic at school, you are required to keep them at home until it blows over."

"Wow, that's good," I said, giving David a squeeze and kissing the top of his head, "because if you told me you were vaccinating David, I would have to kidnap him." Mary laughed.

The star of the household was Annie. I had not seen her in four months, and I was once again struck by the difference in her. She was delighted to see Miles and Laura again, and insisted on sharing their double bed on the first night.

She spoke beautifully, with just a hint of abnormal prosody, a sing-song quality to her words. She and Miles recaptured their special connection, and were so happy to be together that it was beautiful to watch them holding hands as they walked together at the San Diego Zoo.

That evening I asked if they would like to help me make "special cookies," and they both agreed enthusiastically, pulling chairs over to the kitchen counter.

"Shall we take turns helping you make the cookies?" Annie asked in her chirpy voice, with just a hint of her mother's English accent.

"Yes, I'll tell you just what to do," I replied.

When Dr. Rimland stopped by to pick up Alan for a meeting, he walked into the kitchen to find the two children standing on the chairs at the counter, wearing oversized aprons and giggling, taking turns adding rice flour to the mixing bowl, singing out, "Your turn," "Your turn!"

"What are you two doing?" he asked, smiling.

"Making cookies!" they replied in unison.

"You can have some cookies when they're done," Miles promised. "We'll save you some."

"Miles, let me have the big spoon. You can use the cup," Annie said.

"Okay. Careful, you spilled a little!"

"These are our two little dietary success stories," I told Dr. Rimland. "What do you think?"

"These are . . . ?" Dr. Rimland looked at me quizzically, then suddenly he realized that *these* two children had once been diagnosed with autism. "They're—they're wonderful," he said in amazement, taking a step back and looking at the children once again. "Wonderful," he added softly.

Four months later Mary would telephone me with a catch in her voice: "Annie had her formal testing today."

"And?"

"And she does not fall into the autistic spectrum. She tested far above age level in every area, including verbal and social. Aside from her occasional displays of fearfulness, she shows no abnormal behavior. She has no elements of residual autism whatsoever. She is losing her home-based services. *Oh, Karyn, Annie is better.*"

"Mary, I'm so happy for you and Dan. And I know just how you must be feeling."

CLOSURE

Two years ago, when he was only three, I sat in my office off of the living room, trying to imagine how I could ever write Miles's story. By the time I could write a final chapter, he would be in college. There was still so much to be known about autism. Its connections with the immune system, vaccinations, genetics, and food intolerances are still being proven and understood, and will continue to be a source of great debate for many years to come.

Autism is still a treacherous beast, terrible and mysterious. Killing a few of the monsters had not killed the species, only exposed its vulnerability.

But there was one clear reason to write and publish a book about what I had learned so far, and I was reminded of that when a bright face appeared in the doorway. The very sight of it always made me smile.

"I finished lunch and I washed my hands. Can I come into your office?"

"Sure, sweetie. I was just thinking about you."

Miles took my hand and kissed it several times.

"What are you doing?" I asked, smiling.

"Kissing."

"Why?"

"Because I love you, Mommy."

"You love me?" I asked. What a kid. How many three-year-olds would do such a thing?

"You're in a sweet mood," I said.

He gave me an impish grin. "I'm a sweet boy, that's why. I love Laura, too. I'm gonna go kiss her now." He trotted out, calling his sister's name. I heard him run upstairs and then, from the baby monitor that I kept on, I heard him trying to kiss his sister.

"Ow, Miles, stop."

"But I love you. What are you doing?"

"Playing Barbies. Wanna play?"

"Let's play dinosaur cars."

"First play Barbies with me."

"Okay, but I want to be Ken."

The sounds of their imaginative play became fainter as they moved into another room, but continued for a long time, as I reflected on the joy of it.

Eighteen months later, at four and a half, Miles was an amazing, precocious, charming child. His voice had lost its singsong quality and was richly expressive. He was reading at a first-grade level. He had not begun reading in a hyperlexic savant manner but in the way a normal child learns to read—sounding out words in his books in bed every night, remembering the letter sounds he had learned back in those discrete trial drills with Jill all those years ago. He read stories with drama and flair, acting out each character's part. Like Laura, he practiced his reading on cereal boxes and road signs, giggling when a figured-out word sounded silly, constantly surprising us and Cheryl, who had returned to live with us and was now a full-time student at a local college. When Sue came back from England for a visit, she, too, was amazed.

Since he would be too young for public school that fall, we had no choice but to enroll him in a private kindergarten. Laura had just finished a year of half-day public kindergarten with twenty-three children and one teacher. Many of her classmates were still learning their colors when school began, and few had known their letters. The idea of waiting another year before sending Miles to such a class was out of the question.

From the backseat of my car, on the first day of September 1998, he read me the handwritten letter his teacher had sent to new students, stumbling only over the word "acquainted." I had not told his teacher about Miles's history, only about his allergies. I felt my tension over that decision ease as I listened to his expressive voice. He would excel in that "regular" class, both socially and academically.

I was right; Miles loved kindergarten. When I dropped him off in the morning, his classmates leapt to their feet, shouting his name excitedly and pulling him over to join them in their free-play activities. Each afternoon he bounded into my car with the news of the day.

Bonnie Kramer, the psychologist who had given him his preliminary diagnosis, sent her daughter to the same school Miles attended, and she took me aside one day when I came to pick him up. "I can't believe this is the same child," she said. "I've been watching him in the playground, and he's marvelous. He just led a pack of wild pirates over to the sandbox to dig for buried treasure."

"Yes," I agreed, "he's terrific. I don't think people believe me when I say that he recovered, until they see him in action."

"'Recovery' is not a word to use lightly," she agreed, "but you can use it."

"Can I? People have a hard time hearing such a thing. If he is well, he must not have had autism."

When Miles got a part in the class play as a dragon, he decided to write a song for his character to sing when he appeared onstage, complete with original lyrics and music. He sang in a mock opera-singer voice, complete with a surprising, if somewhat forced, deep vibrato:

I've never eaten a princess
I love to stomp in the mud

I've never eaten a princess
I'm so hungry, I probably could!

"How did you write the song?" I asked.

"It was just in my brain, and when I opened my mouth, it came right out."

In April, as the school year was drawing to a close, I had a conference with Miles's teacher, Tom, who described Miles as "a cordial little guy with advanced reading skills and a precocious vocabulary." I told him about Miles's history of autism and Tom was genuinely surprised. He told me several anecdotes about my son's humor and perceptiveness, and his affection for and loyalty to his classmates.

"Sometimes I regard him almost as an assistant," Tom said. "He models a love of learning, which enhances the experience of the entire class. He once speculated that tails might serve as the counterbalance for climbing reptiles as well as it does for mammals. Another time he pointed out that the underlying theme for a silly story we shared was the food chain as it occurs in real life. He can also outpronounce me when it comes to dinosaur names."

Paul Shattock gave a talk in a nearby city, and we were glad to have him stay with us for a few days while he was in town. My children simply adored him. But I was afraid to ask the question that hung on the tip of my tongue. How many people had paraded their children in front of Paul and asked if he thought they looked autistic? What if I did ask and didn't like his answer?

One night I asked Cheryl to watch the kids so that we could go out to dinner with Paul, and at Alan's request we talked for hours about many things besides autism. But suddenly I thought of a question.

"Paul, why do you think Catherine Maurice's children recovered?"

"Ah, that's what everyone wants to know. One theory is that the whole thing kicks off with some kind of encephalitis. Let's say it's the *mumps* from the MMR, and there is temporary brain damage, which is reversible with intensive therapy. If it's the *measles,* the brain damage is ongoing, because the gut is damaged and you have the whole neuropeptide thing happening. Or maybe it's still measles, but something triggers the release of the missing enzymes, perhaps Alan's DPP-IV enzyme, and the problem goes away. This would explain the 'spontaneous recoveries' you sometimes hear about without use of the diet."

"So you do believe the diet can lead to recovery in some children?" I asked hesitantly.

"Uh-oh, we're talking about autism," Alan said. "We need more beer here." Paul laughed.

As it turned out, Paul got to know Miles fairly well. When we said our good-byes, his eyes misted up, and he said firmly, "Karyn, there is not a trace of autism left in that boy."

I was glad to hear him say it. I knew it, but I was glad to hear him say it.

Between you, me, and the lamppost, as Alan's mother always says, there *is* a trace. It is the gift that autism contributes in its mildest form: an ability to focus, a superb memory, a way of looking at the world that fascinates the rest of us. I know siblings of autistic children who have it, and they would never be diagnosed with anything but giftedness. Now that I know what it is, I am grateful to have it in my life.

A good example of Miles's place on the spectrum could be seen one morning at breakfast when he seemed to have drifted back into his own world, with his eyes closed and his spoon frozen in midair. I called his name four times without a response, then again, quite loudly. Just as I was about to get nervous, Miles snapped out of it and smiled at me.

"You know, Mommy, the world is full of sounds," he said. "When I listen to them, I realize that the sounds make patterns, and the patterns all turn into music in my head. Sometimes when you call me, I don't hear you because I'm listening to the music."

I stared at him. "I think we're going to have to get you some piano lessons," I said finally.

If Miles was still autistic, he might also have been listening to the seductive music of the Pied Piper, but he surely wouldn't have been able to explain it to me.

Miles did not know that Paul was partially responsible for his well-being, but the day after he left, he asked me an odd question. "Can Paul be one of our grandpas? I really like him."

"That's a good idea, Miles," Laura added. "He feels like a grandpa."

"Well, you could adopt him as one, I suppose," I said. "He's a special friend to our family."

"He's so funny," Miles said. "I like the way he jokes around."

Later, as I filled out the next year's public school health forms on a table scattered with paper, gazing dubiously at the section that requested vaccination dates and wondering how our pediatrician was going to handle it, Miles came into the kitchen.

"Mom, am I ever going to eat stuff that isn't Milo-food?"

"I don't know. Do you want to?"

"Well, I'm afraid of getting sick."

"Someday, when you're bigger, scientists like Daddy and Paul will find out how to fix your allergies, and then you can try the foods you want to eat."

"I want to be a scientist like Daddy when I grow up. Maybe *I'll* find out how to fix allergies."

"Maybe you will," I said, marveling at his insight. "You would make a very good scientist."

He looked up at the ceiling in thought, then back at me. "Or maybe a paleontologist."

I laughed. "I love you, Miles."

"I love you, too, Mommy." He submitted to a warm hug, then sprang away. "Wait, I want to show you that book Sue brought me. It has my favorite poem in it." Miles trotted out of the room and returned with a handsome book of children's poetry. He leafed through the pages and thrust the book into my hands. When I glanced down at the page, I let out a little gasp of astonishment.

"Read this to me please, but don't read it scary," Miles said, climbing onto my lap.

"You like this poem?" I asked, stunned. How could he have known?

"Yes, I love it, but it was a little scary the way Sue read it to me."

A tear threatened to spring to my eye, and I gave Miles a squeeze. "It is a scary poem," I said, "but it always makes me think of you."

"Why?"

"Because the monster is the way I think about autism, and you are the hero."

Miles smiled thoughtfully, liking the idea. He snuggled in my arms.

"You can read it scary, then," he said bravely, "since I kill it at the end."

I took a deep breath, and let the tear roll down my cheek. "Jabberwocky," I began:

> 'Twas brillig, and the slithy toves
> Did gyre and gimble in the wabe;
> All mimsy were the borogoves,
> And the mome raths outgrabe.

> "Beware the Jabberwock, my son!
> The jaws that bite, the claws that catch!
> Beware the Jubjub bird, and shun
> The frumious Bandersnatch!"

> He took his vorpal sword in hand:
> Long time the manxome foe he sought—
> So rested he by the Tumtum tree,
> And stood awhile in thought.

And as in uffish thought he stood,
The Jabberwock, with eyes of flame,
Came whiffling through the tulgey wood,
And burbled as it came!

One, two! One, two! And through and through
The vorpal blade went snicker-snack!
He left it dead, and with its head
He went galumphing back.

"And hast thou slain the Jabberwock?
Come to my arms, my beamish boy!
O frabjous day! Callooh! Callay!"
He chortled in his joy.

'Twas brillig, and the slithy toves
Did gyre and gimble in the wabe;
All mimsy were the borogoves,
And the mome raths outgrabe.

　　　　—Lewis Carroll, "Jabberwocky"

Epilogue

Lisa Lewis and I continued to run ANDI, the Autism Network for Dietary Intervention, for over a decade, providing support to families around the world who were looking for help with the diet. Before passing the torch to new parent advocates and "retiring" from the autism community, we spent three years writing a book together: *The Encyclopedia of Dietary Interventions*. This was the book we needed when we got the diagnoses of our sons, and I hope it has served to ease the path of new parents starting their biomedical journeys.

Although I have moved on to new endeavors, I continue, as a volunteer, to maintain a website called AutismBiomed. This contains a printable selection of scientific abstracts, all describing the biomedical findings and treatments of autism and related disorders. The next time a doctor tells you that autism is a hardwired brain disorder, send them to www.autismbiomed.com.

My friend Andrew Wakefield became characterized as a scoundrel, vilified by the scientific and medical communities. The evidence was stacked pretty heavily against him, but there is so much conflict of interest that it has become impossible to sort through it all. My perspective, from firsthand observation, is that Wakefield's methods may have been questionable but his intentions were always honorable. There was no hoax, and there was no fraud. He could have walked away when the going got tough, but he believed deeply in our cause. My colleagues and I watched, horrified, as a good man was systematically targeted, misrepresented, and had his reputation dragged through the mud. It was heartbreaking, and deeply discouraging.

In 2005, I sat beside Dr. Rimland in the lounge of a conference center in California. He was quieter than usual. I knew he'd been ill. I patted his arm and said, "We will solve this. I promise we will." We sat there for a while, both knowing that it wouldn't happen in his lifetime. I still believe in that promise, though. Every new study that I find and post to autismbiomed.com adds more pieces to the puzzle.

Bernard Rimland's legacy is a cause for rejoicing. He twice changed the way we look at autism, funded a great deal of useful research, and supported physicians like Bob Sinaiko who stood up for their patients based on their needs rather than medical dogma or fear of liability. Dietary interventions are gaining acceptance, and we are lucky to live in an age when products are labeled, where good dairy substitutes are available, and when our children can receive appropriate forms of therapy.

I realize that so many parents are struggling to maintain the diet with children who are too big to go along with it, with spouses who sabotage their efforts, with other special needs children to consider, with their own life-threatening illnesses to put aside. They are also the heroes of this story, and will continue to be the force that pushes this research forward until the puzzle has been solved.

When I look at my children, at Laura's wisdom and generosity, at Miles's playful and philosophical nature, I fleetingly become the parent I had once expected to be, innocent of the threat of autism, blissfully unaware of how fortunate one is to have happy, healthy children.

Sometimes I do forget, for a moment, but the shadow of the beast has fallen over my home, and my doorway has been darkened by its dreaded countenance. I have grown to care about many other families for whom the threat still remains, and for their children's sake I will not forget the pain, the fear, and the anger that made me fight back. The victim of a stalker probably doesn't feel completely safe even after her pursuer is behind bars. Miles and Laura may both be parents someday, and there is a chance that they will have to fear for their own children. By that time, I need to know that the beast will have been slain.

PART TWO

The Diet

CHAPTER NINE

Questions and Answers

I always joked that I would never get a Ph.D. because I didn't care enough about any one subject to think about it all the time. But because it is about the welfare of our children, autism brings out a remarkable passion for knowledge in parents of autistic children.

My husband can attest to the fact that for three years I wasn't just passionate about helping my son, I was obsessed. But the best thing about an obsession is that after a while you have the ability to describe and share a great deal of knowledge with others. Many people have asked me for help over the last few years, and I am always amazed to discover how many of their questions I can answer. Although I am reluctant to give medical advice, I can usually summarize what is known so far about a specific subject.

In addition, when it comes to discussing shopping, cooking, and preparing for the diet, I can talk all day, boring family members and friends for whom normal eating is taken for granted. For those of you who are as interested as I am in dietary intervention, I hope you will enjoy Part Two of this book. I have tried to include all of the helpful tips that took me years to discover, through trial and error and endless research.

Frequently Asked Questions About Dietary Intervention for the Treatment of Autism and Other Developmental Disabilities

Disclaimer: The following is not medical advice. All changes to your child's diet should be supervised by a physician or a qualified nutritionist.

Q: I don't think my child has allergies, or that allergies could cause autism. Why should I try removing foods from his diet?
A: Although parents have been reporting a connection between autism and diet for decades, there is now a growing body of research which shows that certain foods seem to be affecting the developing brains of some children and causing autistic behaviors. This is not because of allergies but because many of these children are unable to properly break down certain proteins.

Q: What happens when they get these proteins?
A: Researchers in England, Norway, and at the University of Florida have found peptides (breakdown products of proteins) with opiate activity in the urine of a high percentage of autistic children. Opiates are drugs, like morphine, that affect brain function.

Q: Which proteins are causing this problem?
A: The two main offenders seem to be gluten (the protein in wheat, oats, rye, and barley) and casein (milk protein).

Q: But milk and wheat are the only two foods my child will eat. His diet is completely comprised of milk, cheese, cereal, pasta, and bread. If I take these away, I'm afraid he'll starve.
A: There may be a good reason your child "self-limits" to these foods. Opiates, like opium, are highly addictive. If this "opiate excess" explanation applies to your child, then he is actually addicted to those foods

containing the offending proteins. Although it seems as if your child will starve if you take those foods away, many parents report that after an initial "withdrawal" reaction their children become more willing to eat other foods. After a few weeks many children surprise their parents by further broadening their diets.

Q: But if I take away milk, what will my child do for calcium?

A: Children between the ages of one and ten require 800–1000 mg of calcium a day. If the child drinks three 8-ounce glasses of fortified rice, soy, or potato milk per day, he would meet that requirement. If he drank one cup per day, the remaining 500 mg of additional calcium could be supplied with one of the many supplements available. Kirkman Labs (www.kirkmanlabs.com/1-800-245-8282) makes flavored and flavorless calcium supplements in various forms. Custom-made calcium liquids can be mixed up by compounding pharmacies using a maple, sucrose syrup, stevia, or water base.

There are some very good milk substitutes on the market; check for varieties that are calcium-enriched.

Q: Is this diet expensive?

A: There is no denying that many of the gluten-free ingredients you will need to keep on hand are more costly than the staples you are used to buying. However, when you order by the case, the above milk substitutes cost about the same as cow's milk. Some parents report that their autistic children were drinking over a gallon of cow's milk per day but these same parents were reluctant to switch to slightly more expensive rice milk.

As with all foods, convenience products such as frozen rice waffles are expensive, but making these from scratch is easy and inexpensive. Bulk rice flour in an Asian grocery store is about 75c/pound, and Lisa Lewis's book *Special Diets for Special Kids* is filled with recipes that beat anything you can buy off the shelf. You'll find yourself making rice and potatoes more often instead of ordering out. You might even save money.

Q: Isn't milk necessary for children's health?

A: Americans have been raised to believe that this is true, largely due to the efforts of the American Dairy Association, and many parents seem to believe that it is their duty to feed their children as much cow's milk as possible. However, lots of perfectly healthy children do very well without it. Cow's milk has been called "the world's most overrated nutrient" and "fit only for baby cows." There is even evidence that the cow hormone present in dairy actually blocks the absorption of calcium in humans.

Be careful. Removing dairy means *all* milk, butter, cheese, cream cheese, sour cream, etc. It also includes product ingredients such as casein and whey, or even words containing the word "casein." Read labels—items like bread and tuna fish often contain milk products. Even soy cheese usually contains caseinate.

For more information on dairy-free living, there are some excellent books listed in the Appendix. The book *Whitewash: The Disturbing Truth About Cow's Milk and Your Health* by Joseph Keon cites the results of several research studies that conclude that milk is an inappropriate food for human children.

Q: I might be willing to try removing dairy products from his diet, but I don't think I could handle removing gluten. It seems like a lot of work, and I'm so busy already. Is this really necessary?

A: What you need to understand is that for certain children, these foods are toxic to their brains. For some, removing gluten may be far more important than removing dairy products. You would never knowingly feed your child poison, but if he fits into this category, that is exactly what you could be doing. It is possible that for this subgroup of people with autism, eating these foods is actually damaging the developing brain.

Q: Removing both foods at once seems overwhelming, and I'm afraid of my child's reaction. Can I start slowly?

A: Many parents strongly suggest that you try removing dairy first, and then work on planning for a completely gluten-free diet. Gluten can take more effort and some education on your part, and preparation may take a bit longer. Some physicians recommend doing this diet one step at a time to accurately record the child's response and to reduce withdrawal reactions. The experts seem to agree that the milk and wheat proteins are so similar to each other that if one is a problem, the other should be removed as soon as possible.

Q: How do I know if this applies to my child?

A: Although there is some peptide testing available, the waiting time for results can be long, and widespread use of a reliable test is not yet available. The researchers agree that this is a very common problem in the autistic population, so a trial period on the diet may be your child's best bet. Although a lab result is more convincing to a doctor, the noticeable improvement many children exhibit will usually persuade even a reluctant spouse to support the diet.

Many affected children who eat a great deal of dairy- and/or wheat-based foods will show changes within a few days of their elimination. The diet must be strict. Many parents have found that their child did not improve until they discovered and removed a hidden source of gluten or dairy. Noticeable changes in eye contact, sociability, and language are one sign that diet is an important issue. Another thing to look for are changes in the child's bowel movements or sleep patterns.

Q: When my child was taken off just dairy, he improved greatly, but then he started eating a lot of wheat, perhaps to make up for the opiates he was missing. Will I see the same kind of noticeable improvement when I remove gluten?

A: Children who eat a lot of gluten should show an improvement when it is removed. Some parents say that their child's response was more obvious with dairy, and some with gluten. Unfortunately, gluten seems to take longer to disappear from the system than casein does. Urine tests show that casein probably leaves the system in about three days, but it can take up to eight months on a gluten-free diet for all peptide levels to drop. If this intervention is followed by a deterioration or regression (a withdrawal-type response), stay the course! It almost certainly means that your child will benefit. This may seem like a lot of work for an uncertain payoff, but in the lifetime of your child it may be the most important step you take.

Q: The only nondairy, nonwheat foods my child will eat are french fries and chicken nuggets. Are these okay?
A: Chicken nuggets are coated with wheat. Some french fries are dusted with wheat flour to keep them from sticking together. It is a good idea to get used to checking with your supplier or the manufacturer. Keeping a stack of blank, prestamped postcards in the kitchen is a handy way to check.

The biggest problem with french fries eaten out of the house is contamination of the frying oil with gluten from onion rings and other breaded products. Making fries homemade in safflower or canola oil is a good option. If your child refuses them at first, it may be because of what they're missing! Some parents report that their kids have an uncanny ability to detect gluten in foods. Since many of the children enjoy salt, salting the fries might make them more acceptable.

Q: What else contains gluten?
A: Wheat, oats, rye, barley, kamut, spelt, semolina, malt, food starch, grain alcohol, and most packaged foods—even those that do not label as such. There is a lot of information on gluten intolerance because of a related disorder called celiac disease.

Q: After I removed gluten and casein, I discovered that other foods seemed to be causing a problem, like apples, soy, corn, tomatoes, and bananas. I see irritability, red cheeks and ears, and sometimes diarrhea or a diaper rash. I thought you said that these kids don't have allergies!

A: Many do have allergies, or allergy-related symptoms such as hay fever, asthma, or eczema. Sometimes they have problems with foods that are not "classical" allergies and that won't show up on skin tests. In this case, a different part of the immune system seems to be involved.

Q: So if these foods are not contributing to his autism, they're okay?

A: Not really. Current research indicates that in a great many cases, autism seems to be an immune system dysfunction. This not only leads to a problem breaking down casein and gluten, but it may also result in a problem breaking down foods that contain phenols (phenol sulfur transferase deficiency), and an overreactive response to other allergens.

Often, once gluten is removed, this effect becomes more noticeable, perhaps because the allergens were masked by the effect of the gluten. It is also possible that a leaky gut syndrome, caused by the gluten intolerance, is now permitting other foods to pass through the intestinal screen and into the bloodstream. For children who respond to this diet, allergens do seem to place further stress on the immune system, and have often been shown to worsen behavior and development.

Q: But my child's immune system seems to be working unusually well—he is rarely sick.

A: What we're describing is not an immune deficiency, but rather an immune dysfunction. Many (although not all) seem to share a history of ear infections and spitting up as babies (possibly milk-related), or of chronic diarrhea, constipation, or loose stools (possibly milk- or wheat-related).

Other parents note that their autistic children seem to be the healthiest members of the family. In this case, it has been hypothesized that the immune system is too aggressive and ends up turning on the nervous system. This may explain the presence of antimyelin antibodies in some children, and may also explain why some have immune issues like multiple allergies but do not respond well to dietary intervention.

Q: What causes this problem? Autism seems to be so much more common than it used to be.
A: Researchers are not sure, but it seems likely at this time that many cases are caused by a genetic predisposition or by environmental toxicity, combined with some kind of triggering event that stresses the immune system, such as a vaccination or virus. In several cases, prolonged use of antibiotics seems to have contributed to the onset of the disorder.

Q: So, if I can't give him milk or wheat, and if he has some other food allergies, what do I feed my child?
A: Most kids are okay with chicken, lamb, pork, fish, potato, rice, and egg whites. Parsnips, tapioca, arrowroot, honey, and maple syrup are also usually okay. French fries from McDonald's are currently gluten-free (but may contain soy or corn). Certain white nuts, like macadamia and hazelnuts, are also usually tolerated. Other kids may be okay with white corn, bacon, fruits such as white grapes or pears, beans, sesame seeds, or grains such as amaranth and teff (available at natural food stores). There's always something to feed them—even the most finicky kids seem to like sticky white Chinese rice or french fries. Just remember, starches turn to sugars that feed yeast and bacteria so try to keep them to a minimum.

Q: How do I know to which foods he's allergic?

A: Try an allergy elimination diet. For example, keep tomato out of his diet for a few days and then reintroduce it. If you see symptoms, either physical or behavioral, try again in a few days. Try to be systematic, to be certain before ruling out a food. For more information, see recommended readings in the Appendix. Two excellent resources, which are probably available at your library, are Doris Rapp's classic *Is This Your Child?* and *Food Allergies and Food Intolerance: The Complete Guide to Their Identification and Treatment* by Jonathan Brostoff and Linda Gamlin.

Q: I'm already worried about my child's nutrition, and his "allergies" are causing me to further reduce his choices. If apple juice and bananas are the only fruits he will eat and he's reacting to them, how is he supposed to get by?

A: Fruit contains water, sugar, fiber, and vitamins. He needs to get these things from other sources.

Q: I thought the "five food groups" were so important!

A: They are, to an individual without food intolerances. But just as a person who eats a balanced diet might not need to take vitamins, a person with poor nutrition can make up for a lot with a good vitamin and mineral supplement.

Q: So I should be giving my child a vitamin supplement?

A: Absolutely. Look for gluten-free and dairy-free supplements at your natural food store or from Kirkman Labs (800-245-8282).

Because many autistic children have been reported to improve on a regimen of vitamin B_6 and magnesium, you may want to order a supplement rich in these nutrients from a lab such as Kirkman. For a forty-pound child, Dr. Bernard Rimland of the Autism Research Institute recommends 300 mg of B_6 and 100 mg of magnesium per day.

It is likely that in people with a leaky gut, absorption of B_6 (which aids in nervous system function) is often greatly diminished.

Q: What else does my child need?
A: There are six basic things a person needs from food: water, protein (and amino acids), carbohydrates, fats (and fatty acids), vitamins, and minerals (including iron and calcium). In addition, food contains certain phytochemical substances that seem to help with functions like disease prevention. It is helpful to consult a nutritionist about the use of supplements such as Pycnogenol for any child on a limited diet.

Children who have gone for one year eating only chicken, canola oil, potato, rice, calcium-enriched beverages, and a liquid multivitamin supplement with minerals have had excellent results on nutritional blood tests. You'd be surprised to learn just how unnecessarily varied an American diet is, compared with the diets of other cultures.

Q: So how do I know if my child will respond to this diet?
A: The biggest clue is when a child self-limits his diet—especially to milk and wheat. This is no longer seen as a "need for sameness" but as a biological addiction. Children who don't necessarily self-limit but who also respond are those who eat an unusually large or small amount of food. Although the former may not recognize the source of the opiates, he knows that eating makes him feel *good*. The latter may realize that many foods make him feel ill and tries to avoid eating whenever possible. These "failure to thrive" autistic children are very hard to put on this diet because of their parents' fears, but will usually respond when acceptable substitutes to the nontolerated foods can be provided.

Other symptoms of food intolerance or vitamin deficiency are dermatitis or extremely dry skin, migraines, bouts of screaming, red cheeks, red ears, abnormal bowel movements, abnormal sleep patterns, or seizures.

Q: What's all this I hear about yeast?

A: Candida and other yeasts live in our bodies in small amounts. It was speculated that in individuals with improperly functioning immune systems, they could flourish in the gut and lead to a host of problems, including fatigue, sugar cravings, headaches, and behavioral problems.

Q: How do we know if this is really true?

A: We didn't, until Dr. William Shaw in Kansas found unusually high levels of "fungal metabolites" (yeast waste products) in the urine of several groups of abnormally functioning individuals (including people with autism). His first paper describing this phenomenon was published in the *Journal of Clinical Chemistry* in 1995 (vol. 41, no. 8). Since the publication of that paper, numerous studies have confirmed the findings of dysbiosis (unhealthy balance of organisms) in autistic individuals. See www.autismbiomed.com for a list of abstracts.

Q: So does yeast cause autism?

A: This finding may be just another consequence of the abnormally functioning autistic immune system. However, early antibiotic use may actually be the triggering factor for children predisposed to autism. It has been hypothesized that the candida might aggravate a condition of gut permeability (the leaky gut syndrome), which might let the gluten and casein proteins into the bloodstream before they are broken down, so it may in part be responsible for autistic behaviors. Many parents of children with ADD or ADHD as well as those with autism report that treatment for candida does improve their children's behavior and concentration.

Q: How do I treat for candida?

A: One approach is to ask your pediatrician for a course of nystatin, which is a nonsystemic (not absorbed into the bloodstream) antifungal. Taken orally, it works locally in the gut to fight candida. This medication is considered to be safe, even when taken for several months. For a 25- to 35-pound child, ask the doctor for a prescription for nystatin powder (125,000 units per cc) in a stevia base, starting with 1 cc 4x/day. Your local pharmacy probably carries a commercial preparation in a sugar base—this feeds yeast! You can find a compounding pharmacy at the Pharmacy Compounding Accreditation Board at www.pcab.org/accredited-pharmacies.

Probiotics such as acidophilus, the natural bacteria found in yogurt, are other candida fighters and are available at the natural food store in powdered form in the refrigerated section. Some acidophilus preparations are milk-based—be sure to get one that is not! Bifidus or bifidobacteria works in the large intestine and can be of great benefit, destroying pathogens such as salmonella, clostridium, and candida albicans.

Q: Aren't probiotics the "healthy flora" I've heard about?
A: Yes, they compete with candida for the sugars you eat. They are the "good bacteria." You may be aware that acidophilus is eradicated from your gut when you take antibiotics.

Q: That's why you're supposed to eat yogurt when you are on antibiotics!
A: Exactly. As a matter of fact, in the 1950s, when oral antibiotics were first prepared for general use, scientists knew about this candida problem and coated the tablets with nystatin. After a few years, the FDA decided that the two drugs should be prescribed separately (which they never were) and made them stop.

Q: My friend's child tried nystatin and it made him vomit. If nystatin is so safe, why did he react to it?
A: The child may have experienced a die-off reaction to the candida. As it dies, candida releases toxins into the bloodstream and can cause

nausea, vomiting, or diarrhea. It is likely that candida was indeed a problem for this child. Your friend should discuss a dosage change (starting with a low dose and working up to a normal dose) with the prescribing doctor.

Q: My doctor is extremely skeptical. I'm uncomfortable telling her that I'm considering an "alternative" approach.

A: Skepticism is a good thing in a medical doctor or scientist. However, since there is preliminary evidence to support this safe, noninvasive intervention, it is up to you to educate her, state your wishes, and ask for her support. For a doctor it is better to wait until all of the data are published in peer-reviewed journals before advocating a treatment. For a parent it is reasonable to want to help one's child without waiting for all of the results of the double-blind placebo studies. Because this approach does not include any unusual supplements, invasive drugs, or expensive treatments, your pediatrician should be supportive. Explain that you would like to try this for a few weeks, and agree that you will be objective about recording your child's progress while on the diet. It could be helpful to print up and bring some abstracts from www.autismbiomed.com to your appointment.

Q: Where can I find support?

A: Talk About Curing Autism (TACA) is a fantastic and comprehensive parent resource with all kinds of information on diet and biomedical treatments, including a large online support network: www.tacanow.org.

CHAPTER TEN

First Steps: How to Get Started

Because diagnosis sometimes comes more than a year after the onset of autistic symptoms, time is of the essence. If you suspect an autism spectrum disorder, seek an immediate evaluation by a qualified diagnostician, and request a blind second opinion if the diagnosis is vague or unsatisfactory. It has been my experience that when an educated parent suspects autism, he or she is rarely mistaken.

It is unfortunate that most autistic children are not diagnosed until the age of three, but nothing in the current routine developmental screening would alert a pediatrician to a possible case of autism. The pediatrician usually only screens for motor, intellectual, and perceptual development, which may all appear normal until the time at which a language delay becomes significant. However, it is generally agreed that most autistic children could have been diagnosed at their eighteen-month checkup, using a simple screening such as the CHAT (Checklist for Autism Toddlers).

The CHAT was designed to be easily administered by a regular pediatrician during the eighteen-month checkup. It consists of nine yes-or-no questions for the parent, such as "Does your child take an interest in other children?"; "Does your child use his index finger to point, to ask for something?"; and "Does your child ever bring objects over to you to show you something?"; as well as five observational tests during the visit. These tests consist of recording whether the child points when asked—"Where's the light—can you show me the light?"—and whether the child makes eye contact with the examiner during the visit, among other things.

The significance of the test was demonstrated when a study showed that the four toddlers in the test group of eighty-seven who failed on two or more of these key types of behavior at eighteen months received a diagnosis of autism by thirty months.* The CHAT appears to be a valuable tool in the early identification of autism, and it infuriates me to think that it is not a regular part of the eighteen-month checkup, leaving a small but significant percentage of parents to wonder anxiously about their children's decline for months after the symptoms appear.

Phenylketonuria (PKU) is a much rarer disorder, yet it is routinely screened at birth. Why? Because early detection leads to a known treatment. Since autism has been thought to be untreatable, an early diagnosis was considered nonessential to outcome. This can no longer be the case.

With this in mind I designed a poster (page 241) that I would like to see hung in every pediatric waiting room in the country. For parents of children like Miles, public awareness like this could make a lifelong difference. If you would like to participate in the Autism Awareness Poster Project, visit www.autismndi.com for details.

As soon as you receive a diagnosis of an autism spectrum disorder, I recommend that you follow this checklist:

*S. Baron-Cohen, J. Allen, and C. Gillberg, "Can Autism Be Detected at 18 Months? The Needle, the Haystack, and the CHAT," *British Journal of Psychiatry* 161 (1992): 839–43. S. Baron-Cohen et al., "Psychological Markers in the Detection of Autism in Infancy in a Large Population," *British Journal of Psychiatry* 168 (1996):158–63.

1. Arrange for services and order supplies. Spend an hour on the telephone to get the ball rolling. It can take several weeks before your child begins receiving services, and it will happen much faster if you are actively involved. Remember: the diet may take away some or all of the cause of the disorder, but your child will still need intensive rehabilitation to help him catch up with his peers.

If your child is under three, call your local chapter of Early Intervention (call the county health department for the phone number). If he is three or older, call your local school district. If you are interested in a Lovaas-type program (ABA, behavioral therapy, discrete trial teaching) let them know, and find out what forms of this therapy are currently available. Is it home-based? School-based? What are the maximum hours per week that are currently being granted to other children with autism?

Ask for the phone number of another parent who is using this program. If you do not feel that the services are adequate, join or form a parent advocacy group and look into ways to increase or improve them.

If you plan to try the diet, you should obtain a copy of *Special Diets for Special Kids* by Lisa Lewis. The recently updated version includes lots of color pictures and over two hundred gluten-free, casein-free recipes, as well as a CD with the recipes in printable format.

2. Remove dairy products. The moment you have access to the knowledge that diet may affect autism is the moment you should take away dairy. There is simply no excuse for a delay. Until such a time when a reliable test is widely available, this is the fastest means of getting started. Read the "Frequently Asked Questions" in Chapter 9 carefully. Then find your nearest natural food store and buy a carton of 100 percent dairy-free rice or soy milk (remember, not all of these are gluten-free, so before removing gluten you will need to make sure that the brand you are using is still acceptable).

Look for Vance's Foods DariFree, which is a powdered, potato-based milk alternative that is well tolerated by allergic kids. DariFree is calcium-enriched, gluten- and dairy-free, low in sugar, and has a mild flavor that many children will drink as readily as milk. If not, it is very useful for cooking and baking, and will not go to waste. If you like the product, bring the wrapper to your local natural food store and ask them to stock it for you.

If your child will not switch to a milk substitute right away, try it in cereal, or try mixing it in with milk for a day or two (however, as I said, the sooner dairy is removed, the better). Or, after a month or so, try serving it again. As the memory of milk fades, the taste may be more welcome.

List the foods that your child eats that contain dairy. Can they be served without the milk or cheese component? If not, do not serve those foods, or find a reasonable look-alike substitute such as the Ersatz Yogurt on page 272.

Removing dairy may be hardest for parents whose children self-limit only to foods containing dairy. The good news is that these children are most likely to show the fastest improvement once on the diet.

Ingredients that contain dairy:

Milk	Powdered milk
Skim milk	Goat's milk
Butter	Cheese
Yogurt	Casein, caseinate
Lactose	Whey

Eggs and most types of mayonnaise do *not* contain dairy, even though they may be sold in the "Dairy" aisle of the market!

3. Connect with other parents. You may not be the type of person who joins support groups for the purpose of getting emotional assistance.

But banding together with other parents who are fighting for better services, or who are interested in dietary and biological intervention, will definitely benefit you and your child. As a result of such groups, the educational services in my area are terrific, with some families getting up to forty hours per week of special ed.

4. Have your child tested for celiac disease and then remove gluten. Don't panic! This is easy once you get the hang of it. For some parents, especially those who know how to cook, this can be accomplished in a single day. For most, it will take a few days or weeks to do correctly. But the following is a good rule of thumb: *The diet must be 100 percent. If it doesn't say "gluten-free" on the label, or if you have not specifically checked with the manufacturer, do not use it.* Of course, this does not apply to items like fresh produce, plain dried rice, lentils, beans, and so forth. But think twice before using canned or frozen items. See Chapter 11, "Going Gluten-Free."

5. Order the urine organic acids test from the Great Plains Laboratory (www.greatplainslaboratory.com). Call 913-341-8949, and they will send you the kit. This test is covered by most insurance companies and will tell you whether your child has an abnormal amount of yeast in his gastrointestinal system. If so, he may benefit from a low-sugar diet and treatment with antifungal medications or probiotics. Browse through their other lab tests and discuss them with your doctor.

Keep in mind that it is still unclear whether yeast and fungus are actually causative to autism, or are by-products of an unstable immune system. If they are part of the actual disease process, it may be because their presence has damaged the intestinal lining, or because they are producing compounds that cause the abnormal behaviors, or for yet another reason that is still unknown.

In any case, in the myriad of tests that can be done on autistic children, this is one of the few for which the outcome can actually result in a treatment that improves behavior.

For some people with a history of high levels of gastrointestinal yeast, a yeast-free diet also seems to be helpful, perhaps because the constant presence of yeast in one form has resulted in an actual allergy or intolerance to the organism in every form. There are lots of books available on the whys and hows of a yeast-free diet.

The gluten-free, dairy-free diet will not affect the outcome of Dr. Shaw's test, so you may do the test whenever the kit arrives. I do recommend that if you are advised to implement an antifungal treatment that you do not begin it at the same time you remove gluten or dairy, as this can confuse your interpretation of the results.

6. Identify other allergens and remove them. According to the *Grolier Encyclopedia,* "Allergy is an abnormal reaction of the body to substances normally harmless, such as pollen, dust, certain foods, drugs, and insect stings. The term 'allergy' is of Greek origin and means 'abnormal response.' An estimated 35 million people in the United States suffer from various allergies, some of which are mistaken for the common cold."

Although this definition accounts for both allergies and intolerances, using the word "allergy" to describe something like a lactose intolerance is medically inaccurate. When talking to physicians, keep in mind that, to them, allergy refers *only* to a reaction that can be identified by skin testing. Most physicians will admit that certain foods can cause migraines or stomach pain in certain individuals, and will refer to these as *intolerances.*

Although peanut and other severe allergies are often identified early in a child's life, many true food allergies in children are frequently underdiagnosed, and may be responsible for symptoms like ear infections, eczema, and hives. If your child is over three, it is not a bad idea to take him or her to an allergist and do some skin testing for food and environmental allergies. This may also be helpful for younger children, but you are more likely to get false negatives.

Remember, if your child tests negative to allergies to milk and wheat, this does not mean that the diet is not necessary. *Milk and wheat proteins may be improperly broken down in these children, and this problem will not show up in a skin test.*

As for intolerances, there has long raged a great debate over whether food intolerances can cause hyperactivity, irritability, or learning disabilities. Although some labs will do blood tests for a large assortment of such food intolerances, these tests are currently not in widespread use by the medical community, nor are they accepted as standard practice. However, the results of IgG food allergy panels appear to be helpful as guidelines when implementing an allergy elimination diet.

Generally, the only people who believe in food intolerances that result in behavioral changes are firsthand witnesses of such an effect, since large studies have not been conclusive. However, you, as a parent, should make sure that there are no foods in your child's diet that appear to worsen his condition. Until we have a medical explanation for this phenomenon, *you* must decide whether there is a pattern of regression that occurs after eating certain foods.

Milk is one of the most common childhood allergens, as well as being reported to cause many symptoms of intolerance, such as constipation, diarrhea, crankiness, a swollen abdomen, spaciness, a history of ear infections, spitting up, or reflux. Often these seem to be accompanied by unusual cravings for dairy. If milk and dairy have been removed and these symptoms are still present, consider other foods that may create a similar response.

Phenol sulfur transferase (PST) deficiency is the name for the inability to break down highly phenolic foods, such as food dyes, tomatoes, apples, and peanuts. Some parents report that children with this problem also react to foods with salicylates: physically, behaviorally, or

.both. Common reactions include red cheeks, red ears, headaches, rage, aggression, and hyperactivity.

It has been suggested that epsom salt baths should help with the phenol problem, the salts being absorbed through the skin and helping to facilitate PST activity. Epsom salts are available at the drugstore or supermarket, and are inexpensive enough to try for a few days. Some parents report that their children appear calmer after the epsom salt baths, but not after a regular bath without the salts added. (Note: one child I know became unusually hyperactive in the bathtub, and later proved to be highly allergic, in a skin test, to mold. After replacing the shower curtain with a mildew-free brand, the parents reported that this effect went away.)

Many autistic children suffer from chronic loose stools, which, over time, can lead to malabsorption and malnutrition. Check with a nutritionist to be sure that your child is being adequately supplemented with vitamins and minerals, and then look for the foods that are the culprits by implementing an allergy elimination diet. This must be done properly, or you will spend months wondering about the results.

If you suspect multiple food sensitivities, restrict your child's diet for a few days to some or all of the following, excluding any that are known allergens:

Chicken	Macadamia nuts	Parsnip
Lamb	Sesame seeds	Honey
Pork	Sunflower seeds	DariFree (calcium-
White fish	Lemon	enriched potato-
Potato	Arrowroot	based beverage)
Rice	Tapioca	or rice milk
		Broccoli

Remember that the above constitutes a reasonably complete nutritional package, supplemented with a multivitamin containing iron, and the calcium-enriched drink, but please stay in touch with your nutritionist.

After a few days, if the diet has been strict and improvements have been noted, add egg whites (in baked goods or scrambled with salt, or with gluten-free bread as French toast) on an empty stomach, and wait for two days to note any physical or behavioral reactions. If there are none, continue to use eggs cautiously, but avoid using them more than every three days.

The next thing to try could be banana, or apple or apple juice. Introduce as with egg whites, and wait forty-eight hours. If there is a reaction, be wary of introducing other phenolic foods for a while, and when you do, proceed with caution.

A handful of children with this disorder seem to react to rice or potatoes. As a last resort, for children who still seem to display discomfort even on the simplified diet, try removing one of these food items for a few days. If your child clearly does tolerate these foods, you still might want to consider rotating them in the diet (with designated rice-free or potato-free days) to avoid development of an intolerance.

Do not reintroduce dairy or gluten unless you have decided to give up on the diet. You could lose some important ground, especially if gluten was damaging the gut lining. If you do decide to stop using the diet, give your child a full glass of 100 percent lactose-free milk (so that your results are not confused by a potential lactose intolerance) first thing in the morning, and wait for two full days before proceeding further. If there is any deterioration during that time, put the child back on the diet.

In addition to dairy and gluten, many autistic children *don't* tolerate:

Corn	Oranges
Soy	Red grapes
Egg yolk	Colored fruits and vegetables
Tomato	Beef

Foods high in phenols (frequently craved) include:

Tomatoes	Red grapes and colored fruits
Oranges	Apples
Cocoa	Cow's milk
Bananas	

(These should be avoided by children who react to them.)

Don't forget about environmental allergies. For reasons that are still unclear or unproven, many children with autism, perhaps because their immune systems may be impaired, seem to have multiple sensitivities to environmental triggers. Mold and pollens are high on this list, as well as bleach and other cleaning products.

By the time you have undertaken this step, I will assume that you have sorted out many other possible issues for your child, like diet, yeast, and educational services. At this point you probably realize that you are capable of a great deal more than you might have once imagined. Therefore, keep in mind that treating autism biologically is like peeling an onion. Each layer reveals another lying just beneath the surface. You can only stop peeling when the onion (autistic behavior) is all gone.

7. *Try some supplements* that have been reported to be helpful to people with autism, such as vitamin C, B_6 with magnesium, dimethylglycine (DMG), pycnogenol, glutamine, glutathione, and other food supplements. Remember that every child is different, and try to locate a nutritionist with some experience in this diet who can order appropriate testing and make suggestions for your child. Discuss the supplementation with your child's physician.

B_6 and magnesium. Dr. Rimland has heard reports for several years about children whose health and function improved after supplementation with vitamin B_6 and magnesium. Keep in mind that B vitamins are water-soluble, and are often deficient in individuals with celiac disease, so other Bs, such as B_{12}, may be worth supplementing as well.

DMG. A naturally occurring amino acid, DMG is a product of cellular metabolism that has some nutritional properties. It is the dimethylated derivative of glycine, produced in the human body from betaine or trimethylglycine. DMG is present at low levels in some common foods such as liver, seeds, and grains, and is rapidly converted in the liver to a series of one- and two-carbon metabolites. In this form it can be used by the cells to produce other important intermediates. DMG is not a vitamin, since it fails to meet the classical description: a substance that is essential in the diet for the prevention of a deficiency disease. Rather, it is an accessory food factor. There are conflicting reports about whether DMG is mutagenic or carcinogenic, but it has been used for over a decade in Japan as a food supplement without reports of adverse effects.

Parents report that when it works it seems to have the greatest effect on language processing. In some cases hyperactivity can result from its usage, which disappears when the supplement is discontinued, or when the child is additionally supplemented with folic acid.

Is Your Child at Risk for Autism?

- Does your 18-month-old-child's language development seem slow?
- Has he lost words that he had once mastered?
- Is he unable to follow simple commands such as "Bring me your shoes"?
- When you speak to him, does he look away rather than meet your gaze?
- Does he answer to his name?
- Do you or others suspect hearing loss?
- Does he have an unusually long attention span?
- Does he often seem to be in his own world?

At 18 months old, a child will typically do the following:

- Point to objects
- Interact with his siblings
- Bring you items to look at
- Look directly at you when you speak to him
- Follow your gaze to locate an object when you point across the room
- Engage in pretend play such as feeding a doll or making a toy dog bark

Autism is a developmental disability that impairs social and language development. It occurs in families from every class, culture, and ethnic backround. It is not a mental illness and it is not caused by trauma—it is neurobiological and its symptoms can be greatly reduced by early diagnosis and treatment.

If you are concerned about your answers to some of the above questions, speak to your pediatrician about an autism screening.

An Early Diagnosis Provides the Best Chance for Success

CHAPTER ELEVEN

Going Gluten-Free

In this world of convenience foods, following the long list of don'ts may seem intimidating or even impossible. What you will discover, however, is that maintaining a gluten-free diet is really just a return to cooking basics. In general, it is easier to follow a gluten-free diet by using whole, fresh, homemade foods. Cook and bake from scratch as much as possible.

After some trial and error, even the busiest parents will find an easy system of meal preparation that works for their family. The following will help you avoid common mistakes.

Grains that contain gluten:

Wheat	Spelt
Oats*	Kamut
Rye	Triticale
Barley	Semolina

---

*While there is some question as to whether oats grown in laboratories actually contain gluten, commercially available oats seem to contain quite a bit, perhaps because of cross-contamination. Oats should be strictly avoided.

Ingredients that often contain gluten:

Bouillon	Deli meats
Caramel color	Dextrin*
Distilled vinegar and grain alcohol (amount of gluten may be insignificant)	Malt, barley malt, malt flavoring
	MSG (monosodium glutamate)
Flavorings	Natural or artificial flavors
Hydrolyzed plant protein	Rice syrup
Hydrolyzed vegetable protein	Starch, food starch, modified food starch

Hidden sources of gluten (check with manufacturers):

Frozen french fries	Surimi/imitation seafood (contains a starch binder)
Salad dressings	
Gravies	Flavorings and extracts
Tuna fish (also frequently contains casein)	Commercially ground spices
	Vitamins
Ice cream	Medication—over-the-counter or prescription
Tomato paste	
Products containing vinegar— like ketchup or mustard	Candy, chewing gum
	Condiments
Instant coffee	Envelopes
Prepackaged yeast	Play dough
Confectioner's sugar (also contains corn)	School glue

Some people have reactions to the following grains, which are generally considered to be gluten-free. This may be due to contamination by the supplier, in-store contamination, or a food allergy. Determination

---

Dextrose and maltodextrin are usually derived from corn and should be gluten-free. It never hurts to check this with the product manufacturer.

of whether these grains are safe must be made on an individual basis.
As with any new food introduction, go slowly and add only one food
at a time.

Amaranth	Sorghum (jowar)
Buckwheat (kasha)	Quinoa
Wild rice	Millet
Teff	Job's tears

Usually safe grains and alternative flours:

White rice	Brown rice
Sweet rice	Tapioca (cassava)
Potato starch	Chickpeas (garbanzos)
Lentils	Corn*
Bean flours	Soy and other legumes

Avoid canned goods. Avoid prepackaged and prepared foods unless the package says "gluten-free" (*not* "wheat-free") or unless you
have verified through the manufacturer that the product is gluten-
free. Ingredient labels do not necessarily include items added during
manufacture of a product: if the manufacturer buys certain ingredients from another source, such as spice packets, these can contain gluten and be listed simply as "spices, natural flavors, modified
starch, etc."

Because flour can be used to keep items like garlic powder from
clumping, check with the manufacturer or buy spices from your natural food store.

Seeds and nuts can be purchased raw or in the natural state and

---

*Corn protein, perhaps because of its structural similarity to gluten, has been reported to
cause autistic behaviors in some sensitive children.*

roasted on a cookie sheet, lightly oiled and spread into a single layer. Bake at 350°F for 5 minutes or until golden.

Cook fresh, unprepared meats, fish, and poultry, adding your own gluten-free breading when desired. Grind GF cereals in a clean coffee grinder with some salt and garlic powder for a tasty chicken breading. Coat and fry.

Check with manufacturers of frozen packaged foods like poultry or french fries, as they may contain gluten.

Note that gluten-free baked goods are often crumbly, with textures different from those with wheat flours. Binders like xanthan gum (remotely derived from corn, but may still be tolerated by the corn-sensitive), guar gum (from the seed of a member of the legume family from India—may have a laxative effect), soy flour, tapioca flour, eggs, or egg replacer are critical to gluten-free baking. Practice is required—after a few tries you'll know when the dough needs more water or more flour.

Check the library for gluten-free and allergy-free cookbooks— there are many (see Appendix A).

AVOID CONTAMINATION

Use dedicated cooking tools for gluten-free cooking. Do not use the same spoon for stirring different pots. I once had to throw away a potful of rice pasta when a piece of regular macaroni fell into the pot as I was testing it for doneness. Fanatical? Perhaps. But this may be one reason why my son has done so unusually well on the diet.

Contamination can also occur from countertops, nearby open gluten flours, cookie sheets, cooling racks, cutting boards, measuring utensils, and baking pans. Have the entire household wash hands after touching or eating bread. This diet only works well when it is done 100 percent. Gluten-intolerant individuals often seem to be affected by gluten on a "molecular level." Remind your family—even a few stray crumbs of gluten-filled bread can cause a noticeable reaction in someone who is sensitive.

Buy a separate toaster or use disposable foil in a toaster oven. This is also a nice choice for handling the more delicate gluten-free breads. Avoid using your already owned bread machine for gluten-free breads unless it can be thoroughly cleaned. For more information, see "A Summary of Useful Kitchen Appliances" in the next chapter.

The recipe for gluten-free flour made famous by the illustrious Bette Hagman (author of *The Gluten-Free Gourmet*) is as follows:

2 parts white rice flour   *⅓ part tapioca flour*
⅔ part potato starch flour

Add a teaspoon of xanthan gum per cup, and this flour can be used for nearly any recipe that calls for white flour.

Common Pitfalls to Avoid

1. Not reading the package carefully. Many people are so pleased to find a gluten-free product that they forget to check the ingredients for dairy.

2. Being misled by the name of a product. "Millet bread" can be made from millet and wheat flours. Rice or soy cheese usually contains casein (milk protein). Spelt and kamut are other varieties of wheat that are loaded with gluten, even though spelt bread can be called "wheat-free."

3. Not knowing what the ingredients mean. For example, Rice Krispies contain barley malt and are not gluten-free.

4. Feeding the child a food of which he is intolerant because of a fear of malnutrition or vitamin deficiency. All children on a limited or a restricted diet should be under the care of a nutritionist who can

ensure that the child is getting what he needs through supplementation. When this is the case, most parents are surprised to find that a "balanced" diet is not as important to their child's health as a diet free of allergens and nontolerated foods.

I find it ironic that opponents of this diet have protested that it could lead to malnutrition, when so many autistic children, prior to the diet, were eating nothing but macaroni, potato chips, and play dough. For some reason, neither their parents nor pediatricians seem to think that this self-limitation is a problem but rise up in arms when we suggest limiting their diets. It is my opinion that most of the children end up with better nutrition after the diet is implemented. Their parents become aware of the need for supplementation, as well as the fact that the children will often self-limit much less when they no longer have access to the addictive foods. In addition, some of the sensory issues that affected food choices will improve for many kids once they are on the diet.

In any case, after interviewing nutritionists and reading as much as I could, I have discovered that the following are the basic elements of good nutrition:

Water. Make sure that you *and* your child get enough. Many of us know that we should be drinking about eight glasses a day, but often walk around in a partially dehydrated state. If your child has allergies, eczema, or an impaired immune system, it couldn't hurt to use softened, filtered water. If he won't drink plain water, make it a priority to teach him to enjoy it by removing sugary drinks or juice from his diet.

Protein. This can be obtained by eating meats, nuts and seeds, soy or tofu, eggs, and rice (especially brown rice). Most Americans eat much more protein than their bodies actually need. If your child is not getting enough protein, add soy or rice protein powder to his food or drink, or try my recipe for nut butter balls (see page 271). Remember to check that your protein powder is gluten- and dairy-free.

Fat and fatty acids. When cooking, use sunflower oil, safflower oil, pure food-grade coconut butter, or olive oil. I often use rendered ko-sher chicken fat or sunflower oil, although these are debatably not quite as healthy. For those children whose diets are restricted to a few foods, this diet will tend to be low in fat. Children who eat meat and nuts will not have to worry about adding too many additional sources of fat. If fat is low, consider investing in a deep fryer. You can make delicious homemade french fries, which add fat to your child's diet. However, because hydrogenated fats are not healthy limit the amount of deep fried food to an occasional treat. Macadamia nuts are high in fat, contain protein, and are often tolerated even by fairly allergic in-dividuals. (If your child has a true peanut allergy, ask your allergist to find out if any other types of legumes or tree nuts could be okay, but *never* test this at home.) These can be ground into flour for adding to baked goods (adds texture, too) or blended with water into nut milk (see page 274), another good milk substitute.

Fatty acids are now thought to be necessary for several aspects of our health, including brain development. Some preliminary studies on children with autism and attention deficit disorders found them to be deficient in essential fatty acids (EFAs). Flaxseed oil and primrose oil are two of the best-known sources, and these can be purchased in health food stores. I add them to nut butters, pancake syrup, and other strong-tasting foods to disguise their flavors, but some children actu-ally enjoy the taste of flaxseed oil!

Carbohydrates and dietary fiber. Carbohydrates are found in fruits and starchy foods like rice and potatoes. Getting adequate carbohy-drates is rarely a problem on this diet, but if your child is an exception, consult a nutritionist. Fiber helps keep our bowels healthy by allowing for free passage of stools. If your child has difficulty with constipation, consider adding fiber to baked goods in the form of flaxseed powder or psyllium seed powder, which improves texture as well as adding essential fatty acids. Guar gum may also have a laxative effect.

Calcium. Three or four cups daily of a calcium-enriched milk substitute will ensure that proper calcium requirements are met, making cow's milk completely unnecessary to the diet. Gluten-free liquid calcium can be added to baked goods, waffles, or pancakes. I probably shouldn't bother adding green, leafy vegetables to this list, but if you were born under a lucky star and your child likes them, go for it!

Vitamins and minerals (including iron). Look for a good liquid or chewable vitamin that is gluten-free and free of other allergens such as corn, soy, dairy, yeast, and so on. Read the nutrition information to determine if your child's dosage will allow him to meet the RDA (recommended dietary allowance). Buy some with and without minerals to meet vitamin requirements without overdosing minerals. As an example, a child can be given a supplement without minerals once daily, in addition to being given one with minerals twice daily. If your child is constipated, be aware that iron supplementation can make the problem worse.

Fruits and vegetables contain fiber, water, vitamins, and sugar. Despite their nutritive value, if a child is reactive to fruits and vegetables, I have been told by many nutritionists that they can be skipped. Be sure to replace them with a good vitamin supplement as well as adequate fiber. In the interest of relieving stress from the immune system and preventing discomfort, children who have adverse reactions to colored fruits and vegetables should avoid them altogether.

Since excess yeast is often found in the guts of people with gluten intolerance, avoiding the sugars in fruits is another good reason to skip them. When small amounts of juice are used to get vitamins or supplements into a child, white grape and pear juices seem to be better tolerated than apple and orange.

With this in mind, it is still wise to request regular comprehensive nutritional blood testing from the pediatrician. This will reassure you that you are doing no harm to your child's development and will alert you to any deficiencies.

CHAPTER TWELVE

So, What Can I Feed My Child?

If corn is tolerated, you're in luck. White corn chips, popcorn, meats breaded with cornmeal, homemade corn bread, even Kellogg's Corn Pops (it's one of the few GF cereals—but loaded with sugar!).

If soy is tolerated, use soy flour in recipes for really great results. Tofu, soy ice cream, soy patties, soy yogurt—there's a lot to choose from. However, if your child is highly sensitive to milk, use soy with caution until you have established that it does not cause distress or GI problems.

Meats and poultry are great choices if your child will eat them and does not have any adverse reactions. It is theorized that a leaky gut, which may result from gluten intolerance, is less able to handle toxins and pesticides, as well as bacteria. If possible, buy only organic or kosher meat to avoid additives and hormones, and to decrease the likelihood of exposure to pathogens. Be sure always to use safe handling practices and to cook the meat thoroughly. For the really picky or self-limiting children, make chicken nuggets using gluten-free breading, or try a rotisserie chicken from the supermarket. (Find out what seasoning is used and remove the skin before serving.) Hebrew National *low-fat* franks contain soy but are gluten-free. Check label carefully—regular Hebrew National franks *may* contain wheat gluten. Shelton Farms' chicken and turkey franks are nitrite-free *and* gluten-free.

During the Jewish holiday of Passover, which occurs in the spring, many kosher foods with ingredients temporarily free of wheat, corn, and soy become available, so this is an excellent time to stock up on items like cakes, cookies (made with potato starch), kosher sorbet, candies, marshmallows, and jam, or kosher beef hot dogs and other processed foods. Be sure to avoid products with "matzo meal" or "Passover cake flour."

The following is a partial list of breakfast foods that, *at the time of this printing,* are gluten-free. Always check labels and call manufacturers regularly, since ingredients often change.

Gluten- and Dairy-Free Cereals

Barbara's Frosted Cornflakes

EnviroKidz Gorilla Munch

Erewhon Aztec Cereal

Erewhon Corn Flakes

Health Valley Blue Corn Flakes

Kellogg's Corn Pops*

Kellogg's Fruity Pebbles*

Nature's Path Honey'd Corn
  Flakes

Nature's Path Mesa Sunrise

New Morning Corn Flakes

New Morning Ginseng
  Crunch

New Morning Honey Frosted
  Flakes

Perky's Nutty Corn

Soy Nuttlettes

These cereals are loaded with sugar and, in some cases, artificial colors and additives. For a special treat Lisa Lewis suggests that you mix a small handful of one of these cereals in with an entire box of a more nutritious one. Each bowl of cereal will have a few sweet bits mixed in, adding flavor, color, and perhaps more enthusiasm from your child.

Gluten-, Dairy-, and Corn-Free Cereals

Arrowhead Mills Sweetened Rice Flakes*

Arrowhead Mills Maple Buckwheat Flakes

Barbara's Brown Rice Crisps

Erewhon Cream of Brown Rice

Erewhon Poppets (rice)

Erewhon Rice Twice

Healthy Valley Rice Crunch-Ems

Jo-Crisps (made with jowar flour)

Lundberg Hot 'n Creamy Rice

New Morning Cocoa Crispy Rice

New Morning Crispy Brown Rice Cereal

Perky's Nutty Rice

You may also be able to find frozen waffles that are gluten-, dairy-, and yeast-free.

Crunchy Snacks

Even potato chips can be part of a healthy meal—kids usually don't have to worry about fat. However, if your child is sensitive, finding ones made without corn oil is tricky. Your natural food market should be able to order some made with canola or safflower. Again, check gluten-free status with the manufacturer. Also look for Robert's Potato Flyers, matchstick potato snacks, rice crackers, and rice cakes. Check ingredients carefully for cheese or dairy. Lundberg plain or sesame salted rice cakes are gluten-free, more dense than the common store brands, and usually a better value.

French Fries

If you plan to make homemade french fries, simplify your life by cutting them ahead of time and storing them in the freezer, or buy Cascadian Farms frozen organic fries, which are gluten-free. Fry as needed (if you do not have a deep fryer, 1½ inches of oil in a deep pan will work well). Drain on paper towels, salt, cool, and serve. Be wary of fries cooked outside the house—they are often contaminated. However, McDonald's fries are usually tolerated, and at this time are not being coated with wheat starch or fried in vats with breaded products. You must check this regularly, since the fast food chains have been messing around with coatings for the fries to improve heat retention. Also make sure your local franchise complies with company regulations and cooks the fries in separate oil.

Bread

Rice and tapioca bread (available frozen from your natural food store), toasted and spread with nut butter and honey, is a good lunch. Or make rice chapatis by adding a hint of fresh garlic to GF bread dough, rolling flat, and frying in a pan with canola oil. Lots of good nutrition can be hidden in rice bread or pancakes—pureed parsnips or bok choy (white part), chicken, and so forth.

Pastas

Pastariso is a brand of rice pasta that is very close to the real thing. It comes in many forms, including spaghetti and macaroni. You may find that the cooking time needs to be about 13 to 15 minutes.

Mrs. Leeper's makes an absolutely delicious type of rice pasta spirals that contain dried vegetables. This might be one small way of getting veggies into the diet. Cook just until the crunchy texture disappears but do not overcook, and the similarity to wheat pasta will be very close.

Tuna Fish

Watch out for canned tuna fish. If you check the label, many varieties contain caseinate (from milk). If you find a brand of tuna that does not, and have followed up with the manufacturer, you'll be happy to hear that Hellmann's (Best Foods) mayonnaise is currently gluten-free.

Bacon or Sausage

Although you may be trying to avoid nitrites, a small amount of bacon or sausage (Jones All Natural Little Pork Sausages is GF) used as flavoring for steamed rice may be a way to get your child to eat when first put on his new diet. Steamed rice from the Chinese restaurant is a good choice when eating out or doing takeout—most kids will eat it when nothing else is available to them, especially if it's salted.

Sugar

Sugar is really not necessary for good health, and will aggravate a yeast problem. However, in order to get certain foods into a child's diet, some parents have found that the moderate use of sugar does not cause symptoms. For example, if a child with a very limited diet can tolerate pancakes made from high-protein teff flour, but will only eat them with maple syrup, this is probably an acceptable dietary compromise. Joyva sesame candy is high in sugar but it is also high in protein, so this might be a good choice when a treat is required.

To combat a sugar craving, some people recommend stevia. It is an herb that is many times sweeter than sugar, but doesn't encourage yeast replication. It has a slightly odd flavor, however, so use it sparingly. The same goes for pure vegetable glycerin. Ask for them at your natural food market.

Confectioner's sugar usually contains corn, but you can make your own by putting sugar in a clean coffee grinder reserved expressly for gluten-free grinding.

If you decide to use an artificial sweetener in your cooking, I suggest erythritol. Sugar alcohols aren't associated with the health risks of other sweeteners, but they can cause gas and stomach upset. Erythritol, which is a fermented sugar alcohol, tends to be better tolerated.

Flaxseed Powder

Flax is a type of seed, recommended by nutritionists for the fiber and nutrition it adds to the diet. Flax is an excellent source of omega-3 essential fatty acids. EFAs are "essential" because our bodies cannot manufacture them. We must obtain them from dietary sources. EFAs serve as building blocks in the membrane of every body cell. They are a source of energy, insulate against heat loss, and are critical in such biochemical functions as energy metabolism, cardiovascular function, and immune system health. Omega-3s are also thought to benefit those with allergies and eczema. Omega's Nutri-Flax powder adds texture to baked goods and imparts a very pleasant sweet, nutty flavor. Although some allergic people are sensitive to flax, many find that they tolerate it well and that it helps to maintain a healthy bowel.

When using a sugar substitute such as stevia, you will need to make up the bulk that the sugar would have provided. Ground flaxseed powder, such as Omega's Nutri-Flax, can be a good replacement.

Flour Substitutions

Because each flour alternative has different properties (density, moisture content, flavor, fineness) I like to blend different flours into a large canister and use the mixture to replace wheat flour. I keep the ratio of heavy to light flours at 2:1. In other words, two parts heavy flours like bean, rice, corn buckwheat, millet, or soy, and one part tapioca, potato, or rice starch.

White rice flour is refined, but brown rice flour, unless very finely ground, can be gritty. When possible, try blending the two.

If possible, use organic foods. These have been reported to result in an improvement in individuals with chemical sensitivities and are in general a good choice for healthy cooking.

Many children who require a gluten-free diet cannot handle much protein because of issues such as leaky gut, malabsorption, and poor digestion. In addition, many have food allergies that include items such as legumes or buckwheat. Because every child is different, start with a narrow range of choices and wait until the child is stabilized before experimenting with new foods.

For vanilla extract, look for a GF alcohol-free version at your natural food store, or make your own by placing a vanilla bean into a small spice container. Fill to top with a grain-free potato vodka such as Luksusowa Luxury Vodka. Let stand at least a month before use, shaking occasionally. Refill with vodka when low. Keep two bottles—one in use, one gathering flavor.

Yeast

Red Star and SAF brands are reported to be gluten-free. Some natural food stores sell this inexpensively in bulk form in the cooler section. Use ½ to ¾ of the amount called for in recipes specifying prepackaged yeast. One package equals 2½ teaspoons of yeast—therefore, use 1¼ to 1¾ teaspoons of bulk yeast.

Butter/Margarine Substitutes

I've learned more about the harmful nature of trans fats and hydrogenated oils than I ever cared to know, so I suggest that you use the Spectrum Naturals or Earth Balance brands, which are trans-fat-free. Consider drizzling olive, canola, or flaxseed oil on bread, pancakes, etc., instead of margarine.

Substitute ½ to ¾ cup vegetable oil for 1 cup butter when baking. Use canola oil or rendered chicken fat for high heat, such as use in a frying pan. (Don't use chicken fat for cookies—the chicken flavor is too apparent. I speak from experience!)

Gluten-Free Baking Powder Substitutions

Commercially made: Featherweight brand, available at natural food markets.

Homemade versions:

¼ teaspoon baking soda with approx.

1½ teaspoons rice vinegar

Or:

1 tablespoon sodium bicarbonate
 (baking soda) or potassium
 bicarbonate (if you can locate
 a source)

2 tablespoons starch-arrowroot,
 tapioca, or potato starch
2 tablespoons cream of tartar

NOTE: Cream of tartar is the residue in wine kegs, so be careful if grape sensitivities are suspected.

Another baking powder:

2 teaspoons baking soda   1 teaspoon cream of tartar

Mix well. This makes one tablespoon. It's a good idea to make a little at a time since all baking powder begins to go off (start reacting) as soon as it is mixed. The cornstarch in commercial powder helps cut down on this reaction.

What baking powder does is add the acidity that makes the soda reaction. If you already have acidic ingredients in what you're making (e.g., citric acid) you may not need the baking powder, since the baking soda will react with the acidic ingredients to form the gas that makes things rise.

Thickeners
1 tablespoon of regular white flour equals:

1 tablespoon brown rice flour
1 tablespoon soy flour
½ tablespoon kuzu
½ tablespoon cornstarch
½ tablespoon potato starch

½ tablespoon arrowroot
2 teaspoons tapioca flour
2 tablespoons gluten-free instant
 mashed potato flakes (for soups
 or stews)

NOTE: 1 tablespoon arrowroot substitutes well for 1 tablespoon cornstarch.

Xanthan Gum and Guar Gum

Xanthan gum is a must have in your baking cupboard! It helps to make excellent gluten-free baked breads, cookies, and pastas. Used by the teaspoonful up to a tablespoonful. You can generally just add xanthan gum to a recipe if the end product is too crumbly though don't use too much or your result will be gummy. A 6-ounce jar sells for $6 or $7. Although it is derived from corn, it is tolerated by most corn-sensitive people.

Guar gum can also be used. It is said to have a laxative effect for some, so you may wish to avoid this initially. Methylcellulose is a third choice.

Salt, Spices, and Herbs

In place of table salt you can use kosher salt or coarse sea salt in a grinder, since flowing agents containing sugar or wheat are sometimes added to table salt. Buy whole spices and grind or crush, or buy your spices from the natural food store.

Egg Replacers

1 tablespoon ground flaxseed powder plus 2 tablespoons water

Ener-G egg substitute (follow instructions on package)

¼ cup tofu for each egg—good as a binder

1 tablespoon GF baking powder for each egg

1 teaspoon brown rice vinegar for each egg in cake recipe for leavening

When eliminating sugar from a recipe, replace with flaxseed powder to make up the extra bulk. Cornstarch, arrowroot, tapioca flour, potato flour, and soy flour all act as thickening agents.

Some parents report that organic eggs and corn may be better tolerated. Do not try this in an individual with a true egg or corn allergy, however!

Nut Butters

Commercial peanut butter with hydrogenated oils is probably not as good a choice as natural peanut butter, and peanuts are a common allergen, but if your child tolerates peanut butter, use it in moderation for protein, fat, and for disguising the flavor of nutritional supplements. Check that your brand is gluten-free.

Other nut butters are also available, such as cashew butter, hazelnut butter, macadamia butter, and tahini (sesame paste). These are much stronger-flavored, so use cautiously in baking. Almond butter is delicious, but some children seem to regress after eating almonds, peanuts, and other foods that are high in salicylates.

Homemade versions: grind nuts into a very fine paste in blender or food processor. If necessary, add oil, one teaspoon at a time, to improve blending.

A Summary of Useful Kitchen Appliances

The following should be used expressly for gluten-free cooking and should be labeled as such. Otherwise you will risk contamination!

Toaster ovens. Use disposable foil in a toaster oven rather than risk contamination in a crumb-filled toaster. This is also a nice choice for handling the more delicate gluten-free breads. We have two toasters on our countertop—one labeled gluten-free only.

Coffee grinders. A useful item for grinding grains or spices and for making confectioner's sugar out of cane sugar. They cost as little as $20.

A KitchenAid countertop mixer. I had heard that these were essential to every serious cook's kitchen, but I didn't want to spend the money for one (the basic model starts at around $250 and the deluxe models run much higher). When I found mine at a garage sale for a dollar (the cord needed to be replaced), I was understandably excited. Now I cannot imagine life without one, and must admit that I would have paid full price had I realized how often I would use it.

Bread machines. If you decide to buy a new bread machine, look for models with stronger motors that are specially designated for use with gluten-free baking. However, gluten-free bread can also be made without a bread machine, using a powerful electric hand mixer or a KitchenAid. You will probably find that you get better results when you start with a butter instead of a dough.

A Veg-O-Matic (about $20) or a mandoline (a handheld slicer) for making perfect french fries quickly and easily. If you use a slicer, always use the safety shield!

Also, a good potato peeler with a rubber grip is a wise purchase. Pesticides reside in the skin of potatoes and really should be removed—you'll be using it a lot, so treat yourself to a good one.

Deep fryers. Great for fries, and for fish or chicken nuggets rolled in GF breadcrumbs or white cornmeal. Remember—don't pollute the oil with regular gluten items!

Rice cookers. Not a rice steamer. A rice cooker looks a bit like a Crock-Pot and is a fixture in most Asian or Asian American homes. This is something you will want to keep on the countertop. Takes about 30 seconds to set up, and the rice comes out perfect every time, in less than half an hour. Microwave rice cookers (with vented lids) work well, too—especially with premium-quality rice.

Insulated cookie sheets. After all of your hard work, don't risk burning the bottoms of your GF cookies. You'll find yourself baking a lot—good baking utensils are a big help.

Sanity tip: When cooking for the rest of your family, use (healthy) packaged foods when possible. You can buy a loaf of regular bread from the bakery—save your energy for the GF cooking!

SHOPPING LIST

For the first year or so, Miles's diet consisted of chicken, potato, rice, fish, tapioca, banana, egg whites, and honey. Once a week we gave him bacon. We also gave him nystatin, multivitamins with iron, DMG, and acidophilus/bifidus. He drank water, calcium-fortified DariFree potato beverage, and Pacific Foods' rice milk. As time passed, we were able to discover other variations of this basic diet that made cooking and eating easier and more enjoyable.

The following are my favorite foods, which I have used for some time without a problem. However, you may find other brands and varieties that work well for you. Because Miles and many other children are corn-intolerant, all of the items on the list below are free of gluten, dairy, and corn. Most are soy-free or have soy in minute amounts. Remember to recheck ingredients and call the manufacturers *regularly*—ingredients may be changed without warning.

Regular Market

Enriched white or brown rice

Unsalted macadamia nuts (cheapest at a wholesale store)

Honey

Molasses (adds iron!)

Puffed rice

Whole roasted rotisserie chickens with the skin removed

Firm-fleshed white fish filet (great for homemade fish sticks)

Potatoes

Canola or sunflower oil for frying

Halvah candy (made from sesame paste)

Natural Food Store

Try to find a nice big one in your area.

White rice flour

Brown rice flour

Sweet rice flour (optional—use for cookies, etc.)

Rice polish

Potato starch flour

Tapioca flour

Chatfield's cocoa powder or-carob powder (chocolate is phenolic)

Xanthan gum

Egg substitute replacer or Just Whites (powdered pasteurized egg whites)

GF vinegar—rice vinegar, rice wine vinegar, apple cider vinegar

GF baking powder (Featherweight is my favorite brand)

Arrowroot powder (replaces cornstarch)

GF (alcohol-free) vanilla extract

Potato chips made with canola or sunflower oil (soybean or peanut oil may also be okay)

Robert's Original Potato Flyers

Lundberg Farms plain salted rice cakes

Bi-Aglut crackerbread

Edward & Sons Brown Rice Snaps (onion garlic flavor only)

Pamela's GF chocolate chip cookies

Barbara's GF gingerbread cookies

Health Valley rice bran crackers

Pastariso spaghetti and elbows—brown rice or spinach flavor are best

Mrs. Leeper's Veggie Rice Pasta Spirals

Earth's Best Instant Brown Rice Cereal

Lundberg Farms Amber Grain Rice Cereal

Perky's Nutty Rice Cereal (Miles's favorite cereal. Ground with salt and garlic it makes the best chicken and fish coating.)

Arrowhead Mills Sweetened Rice Flakes

Barbara's Brown Rice Crisps

New Morning Cocoa Crispy Rice

Natrol Ester-C chewables

Health Valley Rice Crunch-Ems (contains corn *bran*, which is often tolerated)

Pacific Foods enriched rice milk

DariFree powdered milk substitute (available from Vance's Foods)

Primadophilus for Children (powdered supplement for keeping GI candida in check)

Multivitamin—Schiff liquid or chewables for kids to start out with

Omega Nutri-Flax powder (great for baking)

Spectrum Naturals or Earth Balance nonhydrogenated margarine

Shelton's nitrite-free bologna, turkey, or chicken hot dogs

Joyva sesame candy

Miles's Diet

As you can see from the following charts, there is some increase in variety from 1996 to 1998, but Miles's basic food intolerances remained pretty much the same. Keep in mind that the charts do not include the nutritional supplements Miles received during those times. Although the diet seems very limited, Miles's regular nutritional testing came back without any indications of malnutrition.

Every child is different, so I suggest drawing up your own weekly menu.

MILES'S DIET, JUNE 1996

MONDAY *rice/potato*	TUESDAY *rice-free*	WEDNESDAY *potato-free*	THURSDAY *rice-free*	FRIDAY *rice/potato*	SATURDAY *rice/potato*	SUNDAY *rice-free*
nutty rice DariFree	potato chips DariFree	nutty rice rice milk	sausage DariFree	pop rice rice milk	nutty rice DariFree	bacon DariFree
Potato Flyers or sticks water/DariFree	potato sticks water/DariFree	pop rice water/rice milk	potato chips water/DariFree	Potato Flyers or sticks water/rice milk	rice cookies parsnips water	macadamia *or* tapioca *or* potato cookies water
GF toast honey DariFree	nut butter balls DariFree	rice pasta soy margarine rice milk	leftover chicken DariFree	nutty rice DariFree	fries DariFree	fries DariFree
rice cakes *or* cookies water	sesame cookies (tapioca) water	rice cookies parsnips water	potato chips water	rice cakes water	rice cookies parsnips water	sesame candy water
bacon rice DariFree	sausage baked potato DariFree	chicken (save some!) rice milk	fries DariFree	chicken/fish nuggets *or* toast & honey DariFree	rice pasta *or* homemade bread *or* sausage DariFree	pancakes: teff arrowroot egg substitute DariFree

265

MILES'S DIET, OCTOBER 1998

MONDAY *rice-free*	TUESDAY *rice/potato*	WEDNESDAY *potato-free*	THURSDAY *rice-free*	FRIDAY *rice/potato*	SATURDAY *rice-free*	SUNDAY *rice/potato*
Maple Buckwheat Flakes DariFree	Rice Crunch-Ems DariFree	nutty rice *or* flax muffins w/ molasses rice milk	Garfava pancakes DariFree	Nutty Rice leftover rice milk *or* DariFree	bacon hash browns DariFree	French toast rice bread & egg white) DariFree
potato sticks water	Potato Flyers Pop rice rice cakes water	pop rice water	potato sticks water	Potato Flyers *or* pop rice water	plaintain *or* taro chips water	rice cookies water
macadamia nut butter balls DariFree	BiAglut crackerbread (rice/potato/ soy) diced turkey *or* turkey meatballs snickerdoodle DariFree	rice cracker & salami sandwich gingerbread rice milk	salami sticks potato chips sesame candy DariFree	nut butter & honey sandwich DariFree	fries DariFree	fries *or* bacon "buttie" on toast (bacon sandwich) DariFree
plaintain chips water	rice cakes water	rice cakes *or* rice cookies water	tapioca nut cookies *or* potato sticks water	free choice water	sesame candy water	rice cookies *or* nut butter balls water
turkey meatballs *or* fish mashed potato DariFree	bacon rice *or* waffles snickerdoodle DariFree	rice pasta soy margarine rice milk	chicken nuggets *or* Shelton's turkey dog DariFree	chicken *or* bacon rice *or* waffles DariFree	teff pancakes *or* baked potato DariFree	meatloaf (egg white) *or* rice pasta DariFree

CHAPTER THIRTEEN

Basic Recipes

The following recipes are among my favorites, and will probably help you get through the first few rocky weeks of the diet. I developed some through trial and error or by adapting regular recipes. Some were created by other parents, and some were inspired by Lisa Lewis's collaboration.

It is hard to standardize gluten-free recipes—ingredients vary in density and humidity—and you may need to add more flour or water to achieve the right consistency of the dough or batter. You will have to experiment a bit if your first attempt with a recipe is less than perfect.

SOFT WHITE BREAD

Also makes good pretzels, pizza dough, and challah bread.

This is the softest, most flavorful, most "real" GF bread I've ever tasted, and I've tried many. My family owes my friend Marci great thanks for coming up with the original version, and to Mary Cropley for refining it. This is now the only bread recipe I use.

In large bowl, combine:

2 cups white rice flour	1½ tablespoons powdered egg re-
2 cups tapioca flour	placer (if not using eggs)
⅔ cup DariFree* powder	1½ teaspoons salt
¼ cup sugar	2 packages Red Star dry yeast (or
1½ tablespoons xanthan gum	4 teaspoons dry bulk yeast)

In a smaller bowl, combine:

2 cups lukewarm water	2 teaspoons rice vinegar
¼ cup melted margarine or	2 medium eggs, beaten (or ¼ cup
canola oil	water if not using eggs)

NOTE: May also substitute 3 egg whites and 1 tablespoon egg substitute.

Beat dry mixture with high-speed hand mixer or KitchenAid food processor, slowly adding the wet mixture until well blended. Beat at high speed for an additional 2–3 minutes.

Dough should be soft, but stiff. If soupy, add tapioca flour until peaks hold their shape. Texture should be much thicker than cake batter (does not pour) but much stickier than regular bread dough.

Grease two loaf pans with canola oil. Spoon dough into pans— they will appear only about half full before rising. Let rise 1–1½ hours. Avoid overrising. Sprinkle tapioca flour on top of loaves.

Preheat oven to 400°. Bake for 50 minutes, and allow to cool before slicing. Immediately slice and freeze any bread not eaten on baking day. Because the center is so moist, this bread goes from freezer to toaster and makes *great* toast.

---

*DariFree is a key ingredient here. This is what makes the recipe so good. It is a gluten-free, dairy-free powdered milk substitute made from potatoes, with a milder flavor and less sugar than rice milk, made by Vance's Foods.

For pizza crust, French bread, or rolls

Add additional tapioca flour until dough can be handled. Form the dough into whatever shape you want. I have a lot of luck with rolls or buns—just flatten an orange-size ball of dough. You can also make hot dog buns, pizza crusts, or French bread.

Place on baking sheet, and make horizontal slits on top of your loaves with a sharp, wet knife. Sprinkle the top with tapioca flour—looks very professional and keeps the loaves from overbrowning. Or, brush on egg yolk (or egg substitute and water) and sprinkle with poppy or sesame seeds.

Bake rolls at 400° for 20 minutes or until golden brown. Obviously, larger loaves will need to cook longer.

For pizza shells

Bake for only about 10 minutes and freeze. Defrost as needed, add toppings, and bake until toppings are done. If baking fresh, brush dough with canola oil, put toppings on, and bake for 20–25 minutes.

RICE POLISH MUFFINS OR PANCAKES

These muffins are soft, nutritious, and reheat nicely in a toaster oven. The batter can be thinned slightly for pancakes. Makes 12 muffins. Preheat oven to 350°. In large mixing bowl, combine:

1 cup rice flour
½ cup rice polish (available at most health food stores)
¼ cup Nutri-Flax ground flaxseed
powder
⅓ cup sugar
1 tablespoon GF baking powder
½ teaspoon salt

In smaller bowl, combine:

1 cup DariFree or other liquid (cont. next page)

1 egg or (2 egg whites) (or 1 egg white + 1 teaspoon egg substitute + 1 tablespoon water)	*2 tablespoons molasses*
	1 teaspoon vanilla
	¼ cup raisins or other dried fruit (optional)
2 tablespoons oil	

Add liquids to dry mixture. Combine only until mixed; do not over-beat. Spoon into well-greased nonstick muffin tin and bake for 20 minutes or until done. Remove promptly from tin and cool before serving.

GLUTEN-FREE CUTTER COOKIES

Even Laura, my gluten-eating daughter, loves these—the true test of a cookie. I bake these a lot—thus all of the editorializing.

Preheat oven to 350°.

In a mixing bowl, combine:

2¼ cups tapioca flour	*½ teaspoon guar or xanthan gum (omit for piecrust)*
1 teaspoon salt	
⅓ cup sugar	

In a blender or food processor, place:

1 cup macadamias	*½ cup canola oil*
¼ cup water—more if necessary to remove from blender	*1 teaspoon vanilla*

Grind the nuts very fine. Add contents of food processor to bowl and mix. Roll into balls and flatten. Bake on greased cookie sheet at 350° for 10–15 minutes or until they begin to turn golden brown. I like them a bit golden—they're crispier. I highly recommend investing in an AirBake cookie sheet so as not to burn your GF cookies. Makes 2½ dozen cookies.

This dough rolls out on a potato-starch-floured board quite successfully to make cookie-cutter cookies (dinos are a big hit around here). It also makes an excellent piecrust—flaky and delicious. Cover the edges with foil and prebake for 15 minutes before filling. I always use macadamias—very inexpensive at my warehouse store.

I admit, when I'm in a hurry I just start with the nuts in the food processor, then add the other wet, then dry, ingredients one at a time until I have my cookie dough. It works okay for me, but you may prefer not to cheat, depending on your food processor.

Rolling it out, then flouring and folding several times, then rolling quite thick and cutting with fluted circles would probably result in something like an English scone, texturewise. A few raisins, some clotted cream and jam . . . sigh . . .

NUT BUTTER BALLS

A nutritious snack and a filling lunchbox treat. Miles can handle a combination of macadamia, sesame, and sunflower, but you can use whatever type of nut butter your child tolerates. Laura likes these with natural peanut butter. Sunflower butter is bitter, so use it in small quantities.

To make your own nut butter, grind nuts in a food processor and add oil (I like to use sunflower or safflower) slowly through the feeder tube until the nut butter is creamy and smooth.

If you are trying to add essential fatty acids such as flaxseed oil to your child's diet, get your kids to like these things plain first, then start slipping in the supplements.

In a mixing bowl, combine:

1 cup nut butter
½ cup honey
½ cup DariFree powder

Combine until it forms a smooth, soft dough. Add more powder if too oily. Roll into 1-inch balls and coat with shredded unsulfured coconut or sesame seeds, or GF cookie crumbs. Refrigerate.

ERSATZ YOGURT

Contributed by Lynne Davis (inventer of the wonderful pineapple velvet cake found in Lisa Lewis's *Special Diets for Special Kids*).

¾ cup DariFree powder	2 cups hot water
1 cup unsweetened pineapple juice	½ cup water mixed with ½ cup
¼ cup lemon juice	tapioca starch

In a large, microwave-safe bowl, heat the pineapple juice until hot (not boiling) and stir in DariFree powder until dissolved. Add 2 cups hot water. Stir in the last ½ cup of water mixed with the tapioca starch. It may thicken up immediately as you stir, depending on the type of tapioca starch and the temperature of the mixture.

If not, microwave for a few more minutes, stirring every 20–30 seconds to check consistency. The mixture should be creamy, and about as thick as a milkshake, but not as thick as chilled pudding. When it feels about right, pour into a storage container with a tight-fitting lid and refrigerate 24 hours before serving with a couple of spoonfuls of fruit spread. If you try to use it before it sets, it may be gummy.

DARIFREE ICE CREAM

In a blender, combine 1 cup warm water and ⅓ cup DariFree powder (or use 8–9 liquid ounces of another milk substitute).

Blend well, then add:

⅓ cup sugar

1½ teaspoons egg replacer (or powdered pasteurized egg whites such as Just Whites)

½ teaspoon vanilla

pinch of salt

1 tablespoon liquid calcium, if desired

1 teaspoon canola oil, if desired. Remember, kids need fat in their diet!

Add ice cubes to make 2 cups of liquid. Blend well.

This mixture should be cold enough to use in the ice cream maker without further chilling. Or instead of using an ice cream maker, you can pour it into Popsicle molds. You can double this recipe, but it will take somewhat longer to solidify. Add cocoa powder, chocolate chips, nuts, etc.

PATHIRI PLAY DOUGH

This recipe was inspired by a similar recipe for pathiri, an Indian bread. When making the bread for the first time, I was impressed by the texture of the dough, and inspiration struck. It is the only gluten-free recipe for play dough I have tried that is actually superior to the real thing.

1 cup white rice flour

2 teaspoons cream of tartar

¼ cup salt

1 teaspoon xanthan gum

2 tablespoons vegetable oil

Place all of the ingredients in a food processor. With blade running, slowly add ½ cup of *boiling* water through feed tube until the mixture forms a ball. If dough seems too crumbly, add more water, 1 tablespoon at a time, until dough is soft and firm. Run processor a few more seconds to knead the dough, then transfer to a mixing bowl. Let cool, then knead until silky for 3–5 minutes. Lightly dust kneading surface with rice flour if necessary.

If you don't have a food processor, stir flour with spoon in a mixing bowl while slowly adding boiling water, then knead for 10 minutes.

Store tightly sealed. Refrigeration when not in use is not necessary but will maintain freshness.

NUT MILK

Hazelnuts, macadamias, almonds, and cashews work well. This is a good, high-calorie milk with essential fatty acids. Makes a very nice dessert recipe milk.

Grind 1 cup of nuts in a blender until powdered. Slowly add 2½ cups water to form desired consistency. Strain if desired and save pulp for other baking. Makes 3 cups.

RICE MILK

In a blender, combine 1 cup cooked brown rice and 4 cups of water and blend until smooth. One-fourth teaspoon salt and 1 teaspoon vanilla extract or sugar may be added for flavor. Let sit for 1 hour, then pour through a sieve. Refrigerate and shake before using. Try sweet brown rice for extra sweetness. Makes 4 cups.

COCONUT MILK

Particularly tasty for soup, stews, and ethnic cooking.
In a blender, combine ½ cup unsulfured shredded coconut and 1 cup hot water and blend until smooth. Refrigerate before serving. Makes 1¼ cups.

Appendix

Recommended Reading

COMPREHENSIVE REFERENCE GUIDE:
The Encyclopedia of Dietary Interventions by Karyn Seroussi and Lisa Lewis, Ph.D.

COOKBOOKS:
Feast Without Yeast: 4 Stages to Better Health: A Complete Guide to Implementing Yeast Free, Wheat (Gluten) Free and Milk (Casein) Free Living by Bruce Semon and Lori Kornblum
Gluten-Free Cooking for Dummies by Danna Korn and Connie Sarros
The Gluten-Free Gourmet by Bette Hagman
Gluten-Free Quick and Easy: From Prep to Plate Without the Fuss—200+ Recipes for People with Food Sensitivities by Carol Fenster
The Kid-Friendly ADHD and Autism Cookbook by Pamela Compart and Dana Laake

Recipes for the Specific Carbohydrate Diet: The Grain-Free, Lactose-Free, Sugar-Free Solution to IBD, Celiac Disease, Autism, Cystic Fibrosis, and Other Health Conditions by Raman Prasad
Special Diet Celebrations by Carol Fenster
Special Diets for Special Kids by Lisa Lewis, Ph.D.

FOOD ALLERGIES AND INTOLERANCES:
Don't Drink Your Milk! by Frank Oski
Food Allergies and Food Intolerance: The Complete Guide to Their Identification and Treatment by Jonathan Brostoff and Linda Gamlin
Is This Your Child? by Doris Rapp
Raising Your Child Without Milk by Jane Zukin
Whitewash: The Disturbing Truth About Cow's Milk and Your Health by Joseph Keon

ADVANCED DIETARY REGIMENS:
The Body Ecology Diet by Donna Gates
Breaking the Vicious Cycle: Intestinal Health Through Diet by Elaine Gottschall

THEORY AND PRINCIPLES OF BIOMEDICAL INTERVENTIONS:
Children with Starving Brains by Jacquelyn McCandless
Diet Intervention and Autism: Implementing the Gluten Free and Casein Free Diet for Autistic Children and Adults by Marilyn Le Breton
Nourishing Hope by Julie Matthews

FOR KIDS:
Allergy Busters: A Story for Children with Autism or Related Spectrum Disorders
Struggling with Allergies by Kathleen A. Chara, Paul J. Chara Jr., with Karston J. Chara; GF/GC recipes by Angela Litzinger

Supplements

Houston Nutraceuticals (digestive enzymes)
PO Box 6331, Siloam Springs, AR 72761-6331
phone: 1-866-757-8627, 1-479-549-4536
fax: 1-479-549-4540
info@houstonni.com, www.houstonni.com

Kirkman Labs (vitamins and supplements)
6400 SW Rosewood Street, Lake Oswego, OR 97035
phone: 1-800-245-8282, 1-503-694-1600
fax: 1-503-682-0838
www.kirkmanlabs.com

Klaire Labs (probiotics)
10439 Double R Boulevard, Reno, NV 89521
phone: 1-888-488-2488, 1-775-850-8800
fax: 775-850-8810
www.klairelabs.com

Laboratories

There are a number of laboratories advertising online for medical tests
to check for allergies and intolerances, yeast and bacteria, and immune
imbalances. Before selecting one, check its reputation online and compare prices. Find out whether the tests are covered by your insurance
company before paying out of pocket.

Compounding Pharmacies

You can find a compounding pharmacy at the Pharmacy Compounding Accreditation Board: www.pcab.org/accredited-pharmacies

Scientific Articles Supporting Diet and Biomedical Treatments for Autism

www.autismbiomed.com

Information About the Biomedical Treatment of Autism

The Autism Research Institute: www.autism.com
www.tacanow.org
www.gfcfdiet.com
www.karynseroussi.com

Autism News

www.ageofautism.com

Index

About the Author

Karyn Seroussi is an author and lecturer, and parent of a son who recovered from autism through diet and biomedical interventions. Her books have helped to mark a watershed in the understanding that autism is in many cases a treatable disorder. She has been lecturing worldwide, educating parents and professionals about these treatments since 1996. Her goal is to help parents and professionals work together to provide autistic children with early, appropriate medical care. You can visit her website at www.karynseroussi.com.